"Just as in her blog, Ilana Jacqueline continues to educate chronically ill patients with a sharp wit, insightful information, and, most of all, *hope*. I would buy this for anyone going through life's journey with the extra burden of ill health to give them effective tools and stories that will support them, and of course, a few good belly laughs."

> —**Carri Levy**, creator of the *Behind the Mystery*
> series for Lifetime TV

"An intimate, humorous, and defiantly real guide to living with chronic illness. Jacqueline ushers the reader with intimate and humorous examples drawn from her everyday life—from passing out in parking lots, to the practicalities of dating and managing relationships, to the pain and frustration of relapse and pill diets while reminding the reader at every turn: Never let your illness define you. An important antidote to the dogmatic 'kale and vitamins' tone of most 'self-help' literature."

> —**Alexa Tsoulis-Reay**, senior writer,
> *New York* magazine

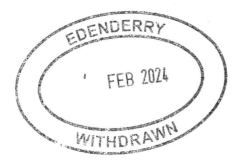

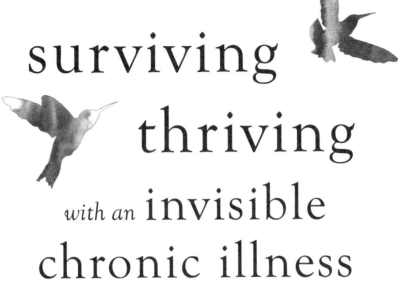

surviving
thriving
with an invisible
chronic illness

HOW TO
STAY SANE
and
LIVE ONE
STEP AHEAD
OF YOUR
SYMPTOMS

ILANA JACQUELINE

New Harbinger Publications, Inc.

Publisher's Note

Distributed in Canada by Raincoast Books

Copyright © 2018 by Ilana Jacqueline
New Harbinger Publications, Inc.
5674 Shattuck Avenue
Oakland, CA 94609
www.newharbinger.com

Cover design by Amy Shoup

Acquired by Melissa Kirk

Edited by Erin Raber

All Rights Reserved

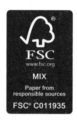
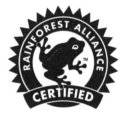

Library of Congress Cataloging-in-Publication Data on file

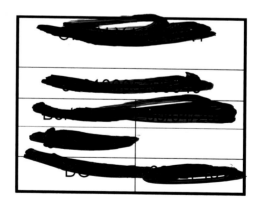

20   19   18

10   9   8   7   6   5   4   3   2   1   First Printing

Contents

Introduction

Chronic illness is kind of an asshole. It doesn't care if you have things to do. It doesn't care if you can't walk down the aisle on your wedding day. It doesn't care if you have to struggle to sit through your graduation ceremony. It doesn't care if you sleep well, eat well, or if you take your medicine on time. It doesn't care if you've got a big meeting in the morning, or a special dinner later tonight.

When you're trying to figure out how to live with chronic illness, sometimes you're going to feel like an asshole too. Like when you miss your best friend's birthday party because of it. Or when you hem and haw about buying plane tickets to New York because you just don't know how you'll *feel* on those days. Or when your dogs or your kids want to play and you just can't.

Sometimes it serves a purpose. Like knowing all the best pick-up spots for chicken soup. Or always having a spare painkiller/anti-histamine/lozenge/sleeping pill in your purse for the friend in need. Or just being the one who constantly makes the whole group take bathroom breaks when one of them has just drunk a 42 oz Gatorade and doesn't want to be rude. However limiting, binding, time-and-energy thieving chronic illness might be, life with it is all about making choices that you control.

Take responsibility for it. Recognize that whatever you do right now is going to affect you later. Know that *not* speaking up and going to the doctor when symptoms strike usually means that they're going to get worse, not better. And, realize that not sucking it up and dealing with it on certain occasions can mean the difference between the people around you respecting you or alienating you.

You should concede that you are one hundred percent responsible for the planning of your future from here on out. Life with chronic illness is about managing expectations while keeping the hope alive enough to still make plans for the future. It's knowing that there is nothing wrong with wanting when there is still the hope of having. As you move forward into a functional life, what will be your way of making money, meeting career goals, and managing your marriage, family, and friends, and most importantly, your expectations?

Me and My Invisible Chronic Illness

Many chronic illnesses are obvious to the naked eye. Assistive devices, such as walkers, wheelchairs, tubes, monitors, oxygen tanks, and other medical devices can be an obvious signal that the person has a disease. However, there are also many chronic illnesses that are "invisible." An invisible illness means that a person can be continuously sick, but may look just fine on the outside.

Most days I get up in the morning and comb my hair. I pick out whatever best fits the description of something that could be both worn walking on the runway and survived unwrinkled while taking a nap. I slide on a little eyeliner. I zip up my boots, throw back about seven or eight pills, and proceed to my parking spot. I get in my average car, wiggle my handicap sign out from underneath the visor, and drop my gear into drive. It takes me a quick fifteen minutes in traffic to get to the hospital. I reach blindly around my seat for the laminated parking pass that reads INFUSION CENTER PATIENT PARKING and throw it on my dashboard.

I walk past the old, the sick, and the heavily pregnant. I see patients whose balding heads tell me that chemo has ravaged them. I slide into a recliner next to a very old man getting dialysis. I see the questions boiling up behind his eyes: Am I a volunteer? A caretaker? Didn't I know that these seats where reserved for patients? "What's a girl like you doing in a place like this?" he asks in a way that sounds more like an accusation than a question.

Having two invisible diseases—primary immune deficiency disease and dysautonomia—makes me a prime target for suspicion. For most of my life, I dealt with doubtful teachers, coworkers, family, and doctors who challenged the idea that my condition was severe enough to inhibit parts of my daily life.

But, boy did it! I had infections that lasted months, digestive issues, migraines, neuropathic pain, tachycardia, chronic fatigue, and hypersomnia. (And, that is just a few of the possible daily roadblocks.) For years, I felt stuck between two worlds. I tried to keep myself looking calm and collected when I was feeling ill enough to be in the hospital. I remember sitting through business meetings with stomach cramps so bad that I soaked the back of my shirt entirely with sweat. I had already excused myself to go to the bathroom three times and my clients were getting frustrated. By the time I could get back in my car to drive home, my mind was a total blank. I'd retained nothing from the meeting because of the distraction of the pain, which added a second level of humiliation on top of my jittery appearance.

There seems to be an unwritten rule: As a professional, anyone can have a sick day from time to time, but you can't have 365 sick days in a row. And, you can't expect every client to have patience and no prejudice in the face of invisible illness.

I'm not covered in rashes or sporting a cast. My illness takes about as much shape as an empire waist dress. My illness doesn't require a wheelchair full-time, but that doesn't make it any less present, constant, or by my side screaming like a toddler on meth that no one else can see. Here are just a few examples of scenarios that I experience in my daily life.

- **Judgment Over Using Handicap Parking Placards:** I couldn't even stand in the line at the DMV long enough to get my paperwork done to get the placard. I had to grab a chair and keep scraping it across the floor. So as far as parking in between those blue and white lines? I'm not parking there because I'm lazy. I'm parking there because if I don't, my system is going to short wire and I'm going to find myself in a situation where I end up passed out near the sidewalk with my skirt up over my head.

- **Cancelled Parties, Appointments, and Dates:** I don't cancel plans because I'm scatterbrained or reschedule my appointments because they aren't a priority. Issues with my health, like the state of my bowels, for instance, end up being the priority.

- **Financial Delusions of Grandeur:** I don't blink at that twenty-five-dollar co-pay because I can afford it three times a week. It's just going on the never-ending tab of medical debt.

I have been through the valley of the shadow of debt. I have paced the hospital hallways looking for a diagnosis, a nurse, or maybe just a teaspoon full of that dignity that got spilled somewhere down that long line of colonoscopies. I have walked out of far too many doctor's offices, fuming, frustrated, and fogging up my car windows as I tried to settle my rattled body and mind around the concept that they say I might never have a diagnosis or a treatment, and in turn, a normal life. When you're sick, the search for that better life never really stops. No one can ever truly "settle" in their search for a healthier, more functional life. Accepting that life with chronic illness is going to be different than what you may have thought your life would be is a huge hurtle, but it doesn't mean you should stop constructing new ways to bring yourself a more satisfying quality of life.

The Blog

It has been hard for people in my life to grasp why I couldn't just "let go" of finding a diagnosis. They struggled to understand why I couldn't just take a pill or shot and be "cured"! I started my blog (www.letsfeelbetter.com) to help those people in my life get the full story, if they were interested in hearing it. Not everyone in my family wanted to listen to what they felt like were excuses as to why my life was littered with doctor appointments and hospitalizations. I was angry and heartbroken by the lack of support from my family. How family reacts to your disease is something we'll cover later in this book. It's a big issue and one that hits hard for many.

To my surprise, as I began to post my stories, people elected to read them! Although some members of my family opted to not read my blog, there was an outpouring of unexpected support from friends, neighbors, old teachers, and strangers. I received many personal emails from readers who were also going through the same issues I was experiencing. Readers checked in as I catalogued my daily life trying out new medications and treatments and hitting my highs and lows of health.

I wrote my horror stories, like the time I had a kidney infection and almost fainted in a discount grocery store because I was so determined to find kosher pie dough that I refused to leave. I wrote about being stuck in the hospital for nine days and having to drink the colonoscopy prep solution every single night because my stomach was so paralyzed we couldn't get it to work.

I wrote about my personal growth too. I talked about signing up for cardiac rehab not long after my diagnosis and going from barely being able to sit up straight without blacking out to walking on the treadmill for an hour. I tracked how the changes in my lifestyle were starting to make an impact on my symptoms.

I also shared the pain of every single relapse. Rereading those posts about my worst moments and how I got back on my feet again took away so much of my fear. When I was having a low point, these posts reminded me that I would get back up again. It's my hope that this book will encourage you to also look back on your worst moments with humor, and to look forward to your next relapse with strength.

How this Book Can Help You

This book will provide clarity in the chaos of chronic illness. Each chapter will assist you through different social, emotional, financial, and psychological issues associated with your disease. Here's what this book can help you to understand:

Even before you can name your illness, it affects your life. The way we deal with symptoms before we have a name for them can greatly impact our self-esteem later on down the road. Maybe you thought you were weak or especially inept at handling life's ups and downs. Understanding that you must acknowledge and accept what you can and can't push yourself to do will help to reconfigure the image you have of yourself.

Know that there is a way to live with chronic illness. Life doesn't end after you become sick. Even if you've been knocked down by a bad flare, you will eventually get back up again and be able to learn new ways to cope with work, family, relationships, and stress.

Throughout it all, it seems like everybody has an opinion. The disease may be yours and yours alone, but the people in your life will have their own thoughts and judgments about how you handle the impact of chronic illness on everything from your daily routine and medication choices to major life decisions. You'll have to decide whose opinion is worth listening to, and whose you should be blocking out.

Your disease does not disqualify you from love, career advancements, or a positive self-image. Once you begin to balance your perception of yourself with the reality of your disease, you'll be able to start making plans for your future. There are tools you can integrate into your life to help you alter your energy level, diminish the limitations of your disabilities, and increase your day-to-day stamina.

We'll be discussing your treatment plan throughout the book and you'll be asked to remember that your treatment is your choice. Chronic illness generally means a lifetime of complex medical decisions. From assistive devices to black box medication, you will find yourself at multiple forks in the road. You'll need to know your own priorities and strengthen your resolve so you can make educated choices with confidence.

This book is not going to convert you to a new religion. It won't tell you which vitamins to take or what yoga positions to pretzel yourself into. You won't be force-fed a new dietary regimen or be prescribed a medication. It won't belittle your small triumphs or shame your momentary failures. This book is a reference for living, even when the world feels smaller every day. It is my hope that it will help you to understand that you are not alone in this battle, and that you are deserving of compassion, love, confidence, and true quality of life.

Find Answers to Your Questions

If the people in your social and emotional sphere of influence have proven to be unsupportive, or if you're still struggling with how to best describe what's happening to your body, you probably have a lot of questions you're itching to have answered. This book will help to answer the following and much more:

- How do you respond to people who call you a hypochondriac?

- How can you resolve the guilt from feeling like a burden in your marriage, relationship, or family?

- How do you explain your disease quickly without confusing or annoying people?

- How do you know which doctors and medications to trust?

- How are you supposed to get answers about what's wrong with you if you have no energy to make the diagnostic odyssey?

- Is this just a phase or are we looking at a lifetime of chronic illness?

- How do you reach out for help?

- What does the world look like for someone with so much medical and emotional static?

- What is there to be done when your medical records could fill several binders, when you've been laughed out of doctor's offices, and when you feel as though no treatment will ever ease the realities of your disease?

- How can you push through when the medical debt builds up and the medications begin to create new symptoms you didn't see coming?

- How can you start the process of organizing the ridiculous mess that has become life with chronic illness? Who can you trust to guide you?

Are You Ready to Get on With Your Life?

For many years, other patients have contacted me through my blog, who are totally consumed by their symptoms and unwilling to believe that happiness is out there for someone who can no longer support themselves physically, socially, and economically. They don't believe that there is anyone who can help them. But, there is: There is always one person left to fight for your best life—you!

Being a patient with ongoing needs, multiple medications, frequent hospital visits, and the responsibility of making life-altering choices about your own future health requires strength, smarts, persistence, and creativity. You'll need to be on top of everything all the time, even when you're under the weather. You'll need to be creative even when there seems only to be one path. You'll need to be strong even when you're past your breaking point. You'll need to learn how to command help, even when you're alone.

Chronic illness isn't something you beat or fight. It isn't a race or a life-long quest to return to normalcy. You don't reverse, battle, or spar with it. Chronic illness is something you outsmart. And that's exactly what this book will help you do.

CHAPTER 1

Accepting Your Life with Chronic Illness

Accepting that you even have a condition that could be termed a "chronic" illness is a hard first step to take. For me, it took nineteen years of bad colds and frequent hospital visits to realize that maybe this wasn't a normal situation. Patients may feel reluctant to even consider the idea that they have a chronic illness because they feel it puts them in a category that they don't want to be associated with. It's a long and lonely road to realizing you might need help, but there's certainly no way to outsmart something if you can't even introduce yourself to it.

You may want to believe that you have a temporary condition. Or, you may expect to find a cure. While that may be true, it doesn't change the fact that until that day comes, you must find new ways to cope. Choosing to respond to each new crisis in your daily life in a comfortable and effective way doesn't mean you've given up on finding solutions to the overall problem, it simply means you're smart enough to want to suffer less. Acceptance isn't defeat: It's a declaration of self-respect under irrefutable circumstances. This is where you are and you're going to make the best out of every moment of it.

This book provides multiple tools to help you to lead a broader, more functional life. It's important to remember that chronic diseases are just as described: chronic. They will come and go, but inevitably, you will relapse. Acceptance isn't about making you weak from the battle of fighting your disease; it's about building a smart and capable foundation from which a relapse can't knock you down.

It's usually best to start with getting to know your disease intimately. The more information you have about your disease, the better equipped you'll be to handle the next move. This kind of information leads to empowerment, and that's what makes you a stronger, smarter patient. Where you once may have felt weak and powerless to your disease, your willingness to accept it and to learn its pattern, and your commitment to prepare for it, will bring you peace. Accept the challenges you are up against and welcome the opportunity to absolutely kick ass.

Is a Diagnosis Everything You Need?

I've been living with a chronic illness since birth and throughout my journey, I've found myself twisted by embarrassment about my disease and shamed about being unable to lead a normal life. I've lost friends, been alienated by family, struggled to build a career, been blown off by doctors, and been thrown completely off course by misdiagnoses.

I thought maybe all my confusion and exhaustion would be cleared away after I was finally diagnosed with a rare disease called primary immune deficiency in 2009 after nineteen years of waiting for answers. When I was also diagnosed with dysautonomia (the dysfunction of the autonomic nervous system), it became clear that while a diagnosis gives you a definite lead in finding the right treatments, the right words don't always cure you. But, having a diagnosis did make some powerfully positive impacts in my day-to-day life.

Validation and Proof

If you can find them, firm answers are good for your mental and physical health. Many chronic illnesses mimic each other. Finding out the exact illness you have puts you on a clearer path of treatment and can help you to find a more specific support group. This was a bittersweet moment for me. I had just been diagnosed with this crap disease, but at the same time no one could tell me I was faking my disease anymore or blame my condition on me or my family. There was irrefutable proof that I had a disease—invisible as it was. It was a real thing and the shame of being called a hypochondriac popped like a bubble.

Research, Prevention, and Support

When you're diagnosed, you can do research on your disease and see specialists with more education about your disease. If you're diagnosed early, you may even be able to take preventative measures to eliminate common future problems for people with your disease. You also have access to drugs that are specifically for your disease, you can join disease-specific support groups, and you can connect with disease-specific organizations and online forums.

After my first diagnosis, I had mildly successful rounds of treatment, but I was by no means cured. Also, having been undiagnosed for so long had created a dangerous issue with antibiotics; they were no longer strong enough to shake some of my infections. My doctors were perplexed about how to handle my treatment and suddenly I found myself back in the game of being a hot potato, thrown from one specialist to another. Wasn't the diagnosis supposed to be everything? Wasn't the chance to go online and learn about what was happening to my body the ultimate goal? The truth is yes and no. For every benefit that I spelled out earlier, there are some drawbacks.

False Hope

Once you receive a diagnosis, you may find yourself believing that your disease will now be immediately cured or go into remission. This isn't always the case and keeping reasonable expectations is something you'll have to manage. If you receive a misdiagnosis of a more common disease, you may end up not getting the right treatment plan for you. And if the treatment plan fails, you could end up feeling more hopeless than ever.

Misdiagnosis

Unfortunately, it's also possible you could receive a misdiagnosis. In a Rare Disease Impact Report published by Shire Pharmaceutical (April 2013), the authors stated that, "according to patient/caregiver respondents, in order to get a proper diagnosis, a patient typically visits up to eight physicians, four primary care doctors, and four specialists, and receives two to three misdiagnoses before they are correctly diagnosed with a rare disease." A misdiagnosis can send a patient veering off into a series of unfortunate directions; wrong medications, dangerous unnecessary therapies, and personal turmoil are just a few of the potential outcomes. For example, they may be misdiagnosed with a mental illness and spend years trying to cure something autoimmune with verbal therapy. Or, they may be given an inaccurate diagnosis of a common disease, when in fact, their disease is rare.

I went through my first two rounds of treatment waiting for the moment that the drugs would kick in and I would instantly feel better. I was hoping to wake up with a different body and a different life. But that doesn't always happen. Years after I was diagnosed with primary immune deficiency disease and the full circle of my poor health became clear, I no longer held the false hope that a label necessarily meant a cure. In fact, I was now having to treat each pesky symptom one by one.

Feelings After a Diagnosis

You may think that a wave of sweet relief will overcome you after the moment you get diagnosed with something, even if it's only part of a puzzle piece. For me, the force that propelled me out of my bed the morning after my first treatment for my new diagnosis wasn't one of overwhelming gratitude. I was bone-deep in resentment and outrage about all those years of doctor's visits, the hospital stays, the invasive tests, and the time wasted. I was angry about how much time I spent wondering whether I was crazy or not. I was surrounded by people who told me I was an idiot! And, I felt like an idiot until most my puzzle came together and I began to find the right doctors, do the right tests, and had a handful of names for the things that had plagued me all my life. Even after the words were there, so many of the answers and treatments weren't.

I wanted my diagnosis to be my cure. I expected my body to change after it came to light. It had been this way for so many of my other friends. A diagnosis had meant a weekly steroidal shot or some kind of treatment and then they continued on with their lives as if they had never been interrupted. Was my situation really so rare? How come I hadn't found the pot of gold at the end of the rainbow?

It's Not as Rare as You Think

A few years after my first diagnosis, I began working for Global Genes, an international rare and genetic disease non-profit. Serving as their managing editor brought me closer than most to the heart of what rare disease patients have to endure before they finally get their answers. Reviewing their stories, I found a few common themes:

- Family and friends felt that the disease "wasn't real" and that hospital visits were often unnecessary.

- Doctors regularly fobbed off concerns and requests for more tests and medications that were very new to the market.

- There was a real yearning for community support and communication both on and offline.

- Patients wanted to connect with other people who had gone through their same journey.

As I edited, I realized that their stories were my story. My story was far from rare, and more likely than not, your disease is more common than you think. Chronic illness is everywhere, and the first thing to remember is that you are not alone.

Make no mistake, the hunt for your diagnosis can be a life-long one. If you've had active symptoms since birth, but have yet to be diagnosed with any recognizable disease, you may be one of the 350 million patients globally who have a rare disease. Whether you've been diagnosed with a classified disease, accepting the notion that you have a chronic illness is truly the first step in learning how to cope with your symptoms and the roadblocks they've erected in your life.

You Don't Need a Clear Diagnosis to Connect to a Community of Support

Many patients who have contacted me from my own blog have said they found comfort in my advice, but that they knew they had a long road ahead before they would be diagnosed. There was a sense of desperation in the tone of these emails. They didn't have a name for the symptoms that plagued them; all they had was suspicion and judgment from their families and friends and painful, boring, or humiliating tests from their doctors.

What I wanted to get across to them was that they didn't need to wait for their results to connect to their community of support. It's those who are in the murkiest part of their pre-diagnosis that often need the most support. Growing up without a community of support, I often went through crises alone. I could only compare my life with chronic illness to the healthy people around me, and that made me feel completely inadequate in every way. Had I known others going through similar trials, I would have realized that my experiences were common and in many cases temporary. I felt that because I couldn't classify my disease, I had no right to support.

No matter what stage of your disease, you are always entitled to support. Don't let the small details stop you from understanding and benefiting from the experiences of other patients who have been where you once were with an undiagnosed chronic illness.

Acceptance is Choosing to Move Forward

At what point in your life did you know that your body was different? That maybe it wasn't going to work as well as everyone else's? That it was going to require you to work harder, be more aware, and experience more pain and discomfort than those around you? Can you acknowledge that at some point, despite knowing *all* of that, you still chose to stay in this body despite its problems?

Can you take a minute to applaud how brave that is? You are among the few in this world who consciously know that they've got it harder but soldier on anyway. Can you take a moment to let go of the judgments of yourself and others, especially those times where you may have thought of yourself as weak or inept? Can you accept the idea that you are strong enough to live this life, whatever it throws at you? That you choose to live despite this handicap? That you know it won't be easy, but you're determined to be in the game anyways?

Believe it or not, you are that person. You haven't given up. You may have made choices in the past that didn't pan out as you wanted. You may have had moments where you've felt like "giving up" in whatever capacity that was for you, like taking painkillers to avoid pain or showing fear when facing a surgery or test. But you're still here in this body because you choose to be in it every second of your day. On some level, you've already made peace with the chaos.

What Does Acceptance Really Mean?

Do you ever feel like you're constantly knotted up with the idea that you must hide your symptoms? Or, you can't let your symptoms interfere with your work, school, or relationships? Are you unable to explain, accept, or even fully believe that your body can't always be as functional as your friends or co-workers? Do you ever get that feeling of unbearable shame when you cancel a night out or call in sick to work? Do you ever see other people at the gym doing more intense exercise routines, watch co-workers stay late, or look over your shoulder at all your friends still sitting at the bar while you head out on your way home? Do you think, "why can't I be like them?"

You may feel like accepting your disease means that you're giving up being a better, healthier person. In your mind, you might be telling yourself: *If I let go, and accept that I have this disease, I'm going to become an invalid. I'm going to inconvenience everyone in my life. I'm going to lose my job and my relationship, and my children won't get the attention they need and my life will be over.*

What if, instead of that conversation, this is the one you start having with yourself: *I have a disease. I have a disadvantage here and if I give myself the right emotional nourishment, internal and external support, information and education, time, patience, and acceptance, I can not only cope with my disease, I can be a functional person. I can be happy because I'll know that with everything I accomplish, not only did I carry it out under conditions that other people never had to overcome, but I achieved it without self-pity or contempt. I do have this disease and every day it's making me stronger.*

Start considering the idea of accepting your disease. Take a moment, and give yourself a break from the shame you've felt, the name-calling, and the frustration. You didn't ask for this illness, but you chose to live anyway. You may find yourself to be many things in this life, but at your core, you are a survivor.

The Long Haul

Whether your disease turns out to be a rare or common one, you'll have to be prepared for a long haul. Treatment isn't always just a surgery or a pill. It is often continuous life-long treatment, medication, or therapies. It can mean making vast changes in your lifestyle, reaffirming your life goals, and most importantly, taking on the responsibility of being a well-informed patient.

Even though you may be looking for the right words to define your illness, your story will be a lot bigger than what is revealed in a single blood test or even the entire unraveling of your genome. I wish I'd known that being diagnosed wasn't the answer to it all. It was the start of the question, "How do I live now?"

Whether you're in your hospital bed, your office, at the park with your kids, or in the doctor's waiting room, the present moment is the time to start cultivating the attitude, perseverance, and knowledge of a prepared patient that accepts their circumstances. It's time to stare down the face of your disease and say: *I know you, I hear you, and you can scream all you want, but I've still got a life to live.*

CHAPTER 2

Self-Compassion and Rising Above Self-Defeating Thoughts

Self-bullying is an unfortunate habit for those who are constantly trying to psyche themselves up to deal with pain and other symptoms of their illness. You might have self-defeating thoughts, such as:

Don't be a wuss, it's just a headache.

If everyone else has the flu and can still make it till clock-out, my pathetic ass should too.

I will not be the loser who cancels on her friends for the second night in a row.

How we motivate ourselves changes the way we think about our character. If you judge yourself as weak or incompetent for having a flare up, you make it impossible to cultivate the self-esteem that you need to deal with the reality that your disease *will* flare up. There are so many challenges to chronic illness. It will undoubtedly bring you through both physical and mental changes: Weight changes, surgical scars, and other physical reminders of the disease will threaten your self-image and how others see you. But, it all starts with how you see yourself.

At fourteen, I'd gone from a size double zero to a seven in the span of two months due to a new medication I was taking. One day, as I was staring at my rear end in an end-of-the-aisle mirror at Marshall's, I said out loud, "My ass is a continent." "It could be worse. It could be a planet," my mother said without sympathy, filing through a rack of dresses. I had already felt like a failure having to go on antidepressants to combat stomach pain that left me feeling like I was constantly trying to digest a sandwich full of shards of glass. Like most women with an illness, my weight was subject to whatever food my body could handle that day. Usually that meant toast and broth, but sometimes it was a slice of cake. It would also vary depending on the amount of exercise I could undertake at any given stage of illness. Sometimes I'd work out three times a week and sometimes I could only work out once every six months. There were times that even walking from the bed to the bathroom was difficult. I was also constantly under the influence of the side effects of my medications. Steroids, a common treatment for those with autoimmune and immune deficiency diseases, usually resulted in what is petulantly referred to as "moon face" due to weight gain in the face.

Over the next ten years, my disease made it hard to eat nutritious meals or even wear a weather-appropriate wardrobe. I think the true test of my self-compassion was deciding to keep my Florida wardrobe (tank-tops instead of turtlenecks) after doctors cut a slit above my breast for a PORT-A-CATH®, placed there for my daily infusions. This meant that I had a huge, sticky bandage smack-dab in the middle of my upper chest. It was visible through all my shirts and without adopting a nun's wardrobe, there really wasn't an easy way to hide it. My body weight fluctuated so much that there was always the possibility that the jeans that fit on Tuesday would not fit again on Friday. As I had begun to accept my body's ever-changing shape, the panic that came with gaining weight eventually subsided. I did what I could, when I could, and I had to accept that some days there just wasn't the possibility of me going for a run or being able to eat a salad. Along the way, I developed my own set of tools, like exercises I could do from bed and meals I could make by triple-pureeing them in the blender.

Over time, you'll find the techniques that work for your body in its worst state. In the meantime, don't feel ashamed. Sick or healthy, your body will go through many periods of change. It's highly unlikely you'll remain the same weight as you were in high school. You'll develop scars both surgical and unintentional that will alter the landscape of your skin. When it comes to body-confidence and the status of your disease, you will soon learn that the needs of your disease will come first. Sometimes that will mean eating a carb-heavy meal when you're trying to lose weight. Sometimes that will mean taking a few days off your exercise routine to let joints and tendons heal. It may not be ideal to have to curb your routine to your health needs, but ultimately you are doing everything and anything you can for the betterment of your body.

Shame: I've Sure You Two Have Met

Chronic illness has a way of killing your assertiveness, stealing your self-esteem, and creating very large voids of depression that drain your confidence and mental fortitude. It's *hungry*, and it's ready to feed on your shame. But, shame is a not a chronic illness problem. It's a human problem.

Dawn Wiggins, a licensed marriage and family therapist, who also happens to be a chronic illness patient herself, explains this concept of shame in relation to chronic illness. "Shame can be sneaky. It tries to tell you that you are not good enough. My personal experience with a chronic illness allows for special empathy and compassion for those who experience chronic illnesses or pain. My own story is one of perseverance, insistence on hope, and a reliance on a spiritual practice. Chronic pain, emotional or physical, can test patients and their families beyond measure, complicate their lives, and get in the way of reaching their goals educationally, socially, professionally, and mentally. I understand and can relate to the challenges of emotional and physical pain, and can instruct and empower patients who may feel their lives will never have a semblance of normalcy." Though it is easy to feel isolated in your shame, it does help to know that you are not the only one. I interviewed many invisible chronic illness sufferers for this book and they all reported the intensity of shame.

Sara, a twenty-three-year-old Crohn's disease patient, and Leanne, a twenty-five-year-old chronic illness patient, both dealt with judgment from their families and peers. Sara struggled to make friends who were unnerved by the idea of socializing with someone with a bowel disease. Leanne's family completely misunderstood her disease to the point that they wouldn't even let her hold her newborn nephew for fear that he would catch something or be dropped.

I asked expert Dawn Wiggins about these cases and the millions like them, and she had some insight. "When we become flooded with emotion, our logical brain has trouble working! The first step is to take a breath and assess our shameful thoughts." In a case like Leanne's, Wiggins says, "new parents are riddled with fear and insecurity and some parents cope with this fear better than others. The instruction to never hold the baby was meant to protect their child, not hurt their sibling."

It's only human to feel shame when we receive negative social feedback. But this negative feeling doesn't mean that we are unworthy. It's just a feeling. The important thing to focus on is that *you* get to decide if this feeling is a fact.

When overcome by shame, the best thing to do, according to Wiggins, is to "take some deep breaths and think of someone you can call or something you can do (like taking a walk, coloring, or reading something inspirational) to help bring you back to a more balanced place. To become an expert in the face of adversity we must develop the understanding and belief that what other people think, say, and do stems from their own feelings and experiences and is not a commentary on our worthiness."

The Shame of Invisible Chronic Illnesses

Okay, so we've cleared up the myth that shame is a solo experience. However, for patients like Sarah and Leanne, feeling excluded can be a huge shame trigger, especially when its related to something we cannot control like having a disease.

For me, living in sunny Florida, my friends always want to hang out by the pool and have a few drinks. Unfortunately, I can't participate in these activities. My condition already creates a general constant dehydration for me, and humidity and alcohol exacerbate my symptoms. I've found myself making up excuses that are everything but the truth. Feeling excluded from these hangouts is a bummer, but I've learned that I've just got to maneuver myself around them. Dinner afterwards? Hangover-resolving brunch the next day?

There are also other shame triggers that can pop up with your invisible chronic illness. Tricia Holderman, now fifty-years-old, had her first ileostomy (a surgical operation in which a piece of the ileum is diverted to an artificial opening in the abdominal wall) at twenty-four-years-old and found herself overwhelmingly self-conscious after her first surgery. "I've had Crohn's disease for thirty years now. I will always have an ileostomy, as there is nothing to reattach my intestines to. I have had a total of fifty-eight surgeries, including many resections, five hip replacements, many scars from feeding tubes, and, of course, this lovely bag on the side of my body."

For patients with chronic illness like Tricia there are a slew of things necessary for survival that can trigger shame. If your experience is anything like mine, you may soon be looking forward to:

- Devices like wheelchairs, walkers, canes, and having to use a motorized scooter in grocery stores

- Surgical scars, visual psoriasis, or other skin conditions

- Devices like colostomy and ostomy bags, drainage tubes, insulin pumps, ports, and PICC lines

- Epileptic helmets, tracheotomy tubes, and special shoes or stockings

While it might be less awkward to not have any of these devices, they are, most often, not optional. Most patients will wait until their absolute breaking point before getting on a grocery store's scooter or wearing any remotely revealing clothing that might expose scars or other signs of disease. They may think that people are staring or judging, or that they're abnormal or different. Self-defeating thoughts like these might begin to creep in. I know I thought all of the following more times than I care to admit.

I'll always be different from everyone else.

People will always see my port/tubes/device before they look in my eyes.

I'll never have the freedom that healthy people have.

I'm not worthy of relationships when my disease means I can't contribute 100 percent of the time.

It's important to begin the process of chasing away these self-defeating thoughts as soon as they come to you.

Overcome Self-Defeating Thoughts

Feelings of depression can pull the light straight out of your world. In situations where your disease has made you feel humiliated, misunderstood, ridiculed, and abnormal, your thoughts may go right to the worst conclusions. If you start to catch yourself thinking some of the phrases above, try to reason with yourself. Don't validate absolute statements with reasoning; "always" and "never" are not *always* the case. You are not "always" inconveniencing people. You are not "never" feeling well enough to see your friends. You may just be having a particularly bad flare up.

Remember Who You Really Are

Why such a silly statement? Because when a disease feels like it's started to take over your body, you must consciously, forcefully, and repetitively remind yourself that you are still the person you were before disease. The disease is not *all* of what makes up your character. Remind yourself of your positive qualities. While other people's first impressions may misalign with what is true, it doesn't mean a chance to have a connection with them is ruined. There will always be time to change another person's perception of you. If you know who you are, communicating your truth with new people will come easily.

Stand Up for Yourself

Stand up for yourself when someone tries to knock you down or makes you feel unworthy. However, the person you'll fight the most emotional battles with is you. You must be your own personal advocate. Don't be a bully to your own subconscious.

27

Coping with Body Shame

Once you've been diagnosed with a serious disease, the relationship to your body can be profoundly altered. After discussing the topic of body shame with several patients and mental health professionals over the course of my illness, I learned that there are some coping mechanisms you can use to deal with your mind-set around sudden or gradual physical changes. Kait Scalisi, a sex educator who works with chronic illness patients, provides some strategies for responding to the psychological impact of how chronic illness affects our bodies and how we feel about their worth during sickness.

> **Focus on the Positive:** The first strategy she suggests is to begin by focusing on the things you do like about your body. This can be especially challenging for a population of patients who spend most of their days just trying to get their body's tantrums to quiet down long enough to get through one activity and on to the next. Start naming parts of your body that you're grateful for. Not just aesthetics either. Can you eat today? Can you walk? Can you see clearly?

> **Get Naked:** Get familiar with your body. It's a good rule to be aware enough of your body to know when serious changes have occurred. It's also useful to familiarize and get comfortable with your physical frame. Face the changes head-on each day.

> **Find Your Role Models:** Okay, so we can probably cross Tyra Banks off the list, but there are plenty of men and women whose bodies are beautiful even though they're not the norm. Find inspiration in the stories of patients running marathons to raise funds for their own treatment,

wearing bathing suits in public despite having visual medical devices, and even going into careers as professional models for their unique and inspiring appeal.

The key to body confidence for Scalisi is that you "focus on all the things your body can do." The operative word is *can*. Scalisi says, "Perhaps you have gained weight but still can inspire a room with your voice. Perhaps you're in a wheelchair but the best cook on the block. Perhaps you have surgical scars or an ostomy bag but can still teach your favorite fitness class. Such thinking helps put the changes you're experiencing, which can sometimes feel overwhelming, into perspective."

Cultivating a New Attitude Away from Shame

It can be difficult to learn to love the invisible and visible scars of your disease and not be ashamed of them and your body. Scars can be terrible reminders of the pain you experienced, but they can also be reminders of having overcome. After my first abdominal surgery, I would look down at my body in the bathtub and just cry. My scars had healed into raised, keloid mounds and there were just so many of them. I could never wear a bikini again! But over the next few months, as I experienced unimaginable relief from my surgery, I realized that my scars were a small price to pay to be able to eat, to have more energy, and to experience so much less pain than before. They became symbols of strength to me. And when it was time for the next surgery, I met my recovery with the confidence that any imperfection on the inside was worth whatever reflection on the outside.

Although Travis Love, thirty-years-old, suffered from shameful thoughts about his chronic illness, he was also able to cultivate new ways of thinking about the scars of his disease. At seventeen years old, he had two scars because of doctors failing to install a life-saving device on one side of his chest on their first try. "I have two scars and a bump where the port is now," explains Travis. "What's worse is that they installed one size larger, thinking that my body would grow into it and it never did. But, when they were implanting the port, they fixed the hernia and I finally had a stomach to show off. I was tired of hiding, so most of that first summer I walked around the house without a shirt, just getting used to the concept, until one day I answered the door without thinking about it." What sets Travis apart and makes him a great example of how we can fight back against our self-defeating thoughts is his attitude.

As Scalsi mentions, getting used to one's bare appearance can encourage approval about your body. This is not to say that Travis was never self-conscious about his body or port from then on, but his attitude of flexibility and non-judgment helped drive his decisions about how he wanted to treat his body. To cover up one of the scars on his left chest muscle, he got a tattoo there and on his arm. He explains that these have been great talking pieces, as well as an easy distraction from his port when summer comes around, because they "stand out quite a bit in contrast to my ghostly white skin."

Travis has always had his positive attitude to fall back on. Admittedly, some of us don't, which can mean your self-esteem can sometimes take a beating. If this is the case, it's important to try and cultivate an attitude to combat these feelings:

Know your limits. If your symptoms are flaring up, it might not be the time to vigorously exercise. Rest when you need it even if you're worried you'll be judged as lazy.

Know that change is inevitable. Even if you didn't have a chronic illness, you probably wouldn't have gone on to have a size zero wardrobe past puberty. We are always changing, sometimes we even go back to the way we were before.

Know that life goes on. You may now have to get around the grocery store in one of those scooters, but you still must pick up pop-tarts. Don't be embarrassed when you need to mobilize yourself in a new way.

Know you're never alone. Man or woman, young or old, sick or well—we all have deep psychological scars. "We are the only thinkers in our minds. What you think about yourself will dictate how much or little what others think affects you," Dawn Wiggins reminds us. "We get to decide if our diagnosis is going to steal our joy, identity, determination, our compassion and empathy for others, and most importantly our worthiness." It won't happen overnight, but making time and focusing on accepting your imperfections is as important as any other pill you'll have to swallow.

Tell Your Story

Though it is important to seek the opinion and counsel of experts, in my research for this book, I heard several self-soothing ideas that help to fight against the shame monster. Though I heard similar sounding ideas from many others, Tricia summed them up beautifully: "One of the things that helped me the most was talking to young girls and women who were about to have the surgery I had. I realized how much better life and living were after the surgery."

Telling your story in all forms, whether spoken as a mentor, written online, or communicated to a friend, can be a strong tool for healing and can help you make sense of some of the conflicting feelings you might have about your disease. Yes, you may have garnered some unwanted results, you may still feel separated from the norm, but for the most part, has your life improved with treatment? What have you learned about your personal character and strength through your journey?

"My advice," Tricia continues, "would be to respect the needs of your body first." Regularly, we're faced with two options: fight and conceal what we feel to be embarrassing symptoms or accept and explain our disease to ourselves and others. By honoring these self-defeating thoughts of *I'm not good enough, I'm not normal enough, I'm not beautiful the way I am, I'm unlovable, my disease is all I am,* we encourage ourselves to crawl deeper into depression, anxiety, and isolation.

Practice Positive Thinking

It's only natural to have moments of self-doubt when it comes to our appearance. We can't look perfect in every photo. We won't look perfect in every outfit we try on. Coming to peace with your body doesn't mean feeling entirely and completely satisfied with your appearance. It means you have accepted the reality that, at the moment, your physical health is more important than your vanity. Here are some tools to practice positive thinking when self-doubt creeps in.

Find an outlet to express and challenge negative thoughts. For me, it was blogging. I needed to write down my daily experiences so I could remember the good days and know that I was not *always* unavailable to my friends and family. You may want to do the same. You could take up photography to capture the great things in life, or take on other creative projects that can help you compile the positive points in your life.

Be at peace with your appearance. As I've already discussed, sometimes all it takes is a regular good look in the mirror. You may want to make a list of the parts of your body that you love or the sports, activities, or talents that make your body unique. You may also want to put the clothes that you no longer feel look good on you into storage for a while. Maybe they'll look good again in the future, but they shouldn't be hanging in your closet as a daily reminder of where you no longer are. Start dressing for the body you have and you'll experience less internal self-doubt over your appearance.

You could also utilize other ways to highlight your best features. Change your make-up routine. Find new fitness routines that you can manage that may focus on areas of your body that are not affected by your disease. (For instance, you may have arthritic joints in your knees, but you're still able to do upper-body work outs.) You can focus more of your attention on toning your arms than on worrying about wearing short shorts.

Look in the Mirror with Fresh Eyes

I still have my running shoes by the door. I didn't stop buying clothes that both comforted and flattered me. And even on my ugliest days I make the effort to look myself in the mirror and try my best to laugh. *So, this may not be the best day for my glamour shots,* I think, *but I can't compare pictures of my friends at parties on Facebook to what I'm seeing in the mirror this morning.* Our bodies are running through two entirely different worlds. It's in the comparison of those two worlds that compassion can get lost.

In this chapter, we've discussed the shame we feel about how we see ourselves and how we feel others perceive us. We've considered how focusing on the positive and familiarizing ourselves with our new bodies can help us cope with bodily shame. And, lastly, we've discussed how to cultivate a new attitude to increase confidence and acceptance.

It's never too late to start looking in the mirror with fresh eyes. Practice positive self-talk and take the bullying down a notch. In the next chapter, we'll explore how others may react and respond to your illness and just how much your attitude about your disease plays a role in that.

CHAPTER 3

What They're Going to Say About You

Most people in your life may feel inconvenienced by your chronic illness. To them, the solution seems simple: just stop being sick! They may think of you as lazy, attention-seeking, weak-willed, or reckless. These perceptions seem to always be present in interactions with friends and family and are reinforced when you need to cancel plans, can't make family dinners, or need to head home early from work. The pressure of committing to events is raised ten-fold. Will you be accused of being selfish if you need to cancel or back out? Will they think you're uninterested or too good for their company?

In this chapter, we're going to discuss your relationships with other people, how your disease affects your social life, and how to use tools to handle miscommunications about your symptoms. We'll explore how your disease informs the realities of your relationships and map out why those people in your life may not be ready to handle your situation. We'll offer useful tools for opening the conversation and clearing the air, as well as helping you to determine which people you should be surrounding yourself with and who it's time to take a break from.

The Realities of Your Relationships

A few years ago, I started following this woman Ally on Facebook. She was always in the hospital, and at the time, so was I. While I grumbled and bitched about the cold rooms and invasive procedures, Ally was literally having her head drained of spinal fluid day after day, with a smile on.

Ally had been diagnosed with intracranial hypotension. As limiting as her outcome looked, and as often as she had to shave her head for brain surgery, she remained positive, almost mocking it in her own determinedly cheerful way. She would share pictures of her head in bandages, the piles of life-sustaining machinery surrounding her, and Disney princess coloring books and handmade blankets that her nurses or friends had made for her.

But I would always wonder, where is Ally's family? The answer was disappointing, but not surprising. "Before my diagnoses, everybody thought I was faking it," said Ally. Despite her constant headaches and vomiting, dizziness and balance issues, she struggled to obtain their support. Her mother wasn't interested in helping her find answers from her local teaching hospital. She was only interested in taking Ally for alternative therapies, fearing any more complicated treatment might injure her further. The rest of her family failed to understand her condition as well. The constant comments included: "I wish I had a headache so I could stay home all day," or "If you wouldn't pass out all the time I wouldn't be embarrassed to go out with you."

It's not entirely surprising to see family members react to a diagnosis of an invisible disease with insensitive comments like these. Like Ally's family, many can only make sense of the peripheral "perks" of disease. When they don't see a condition as valid, they feel as though someone is taking handicapped privileges and exploiting them, and they feel the need to react accordingly. Sometimes the reactions are in the form of accusatory comments or ignoring the person in pain, and sometimes the interactions lead to hostility and fighting.

Education will be your best and sometimes only tool in these cases. Dragging family or friends to doctor appointments and hospital stays and printing out literature from a disease organization's website can give you a chance to start a conversation about your illness with them. Discussing how the disease affects the body, the long-term outlook of the condition, and what other patients in similar situations have done will help your loved ones better understand how they can support you.

Unfortunately, Ally did not receive the support she needed from her parents. She said, "Once I finally had my first diagnosis, my mom did a little bit of research, but still was only interested in alternative therapy until the doctors told her it needed to be handled differently. Still to this day my dad isn't aware of all the diseases I face, or the treatments I do. He still makes rude comments telling me how lazy I am and how disappointed he is." Ally still wants support from her parents, especially during difficult surgeries and debilitating flares, but she understands that because her parents have never experienced anything like her health issues, they may not ever have the capacity to empathize.

There are many patients out there who will never feel completely supported by family and friends. That great pillar of strength that's supposed to help you through the hard times may not be there at the time your first symptoms hit. As you grow and learn more about yourself and your disease, you'll be able to build your support system. Ally began to befriend student nurses who often worked with her doctors. She became a regular at the hospital and consequently found that her family of support was the hospital staff. She continued to grow support by making friends online and through her school. In the absence of her family's understanding of her disease, Ally managed to create a wonderful team of support. We cannot back down from the idea that we are deserving of support and understanding in our time of need, but the reality is we might not get it from the people we expect it from.

Dawn Wiggins, the licensed marriage and family therapist from chapter one, shed some light on why Ally's family had difficulty coping with her disease. "For Ally, I would guess that the reason behind her unsupportive family not giving her the support she wants or needs is about feelings of powerlessness," says Wiggins. "In my experience, most loved ones just want to solve the problem. When families don't understand the illness and when medical science has a difficult time understanding and treating that condition, it leads to a feeling of powerlessness. Powerlessness is such a strong and uncomfortable feeling that many will do anything they can to avoid it."

So how can you tell if your family members or friends are feeling powerless? Wiggins says some clues this may be the case is when they are acting like they have the solution, try to control the situation, or are pushing their feelings onto someone else, like the patient or their spouse. These feelings and behaviors can ultimately cause some painful conversations, accusations, and an erosion of crucial relationships. In these cases, well-meaning family members end up hurting the people they care most about. For Wiggins, the first step in this situation is similar to what we covered in chapter one: "Most patients just want to be heard and reassured that our lives aren't going to end as a result of our illness. My professional suggestion to caretakers and loved ones is to focus on acceptance of the circumstances as they are today and to understand that healing is a process, a continuous one."

As we have learned in the last two chapters, acceptance is something that you need to cultivate as well. You are the ultimate model for how people will treat you and your situation. The following are some tips for when a well-meaning person tries to help, but unwittingly provokes your anger and frustration by thinking they can solve a problem you can't.

- Recognize this isn't a personal attack; they are trying to help in the only way they know how.

- Acknowledge their support while politely letting them know that the way they're going about it is ineffective.

- Give them ways in which they *can* help. For example, helping you get to the doctor, going on a disease organization's website and reading up on the facts, and simply being there to support you emotionally during procedures or other moments when you're in need.

Unease About Your Disease

Even my mother, my greatest supporter, at times felt her own sense of powerlessness to assist me. She told me that once when she was thinking that there must be something more to this that I wasn't telling her, she rifled through my drawers and swiped her hands under my mattress looking for empty packets of laxatives. This kind of thinking was something I was often faced with. People would say:

She's probably taking diet pills.

You don't just have excruciating stomach pain for no reason.

How many scopes has she had at this point? Ten? And they've found nothing?

I can always remember my mom advocating for me, but there were moments I saw her doubt her own resolve. Maybe these symptoms *were* just psychological. She had to do something! In addition to all my specialists, she took me to acupuncturists, herbalists, chiropractors, and a series of psychologists and psychiatrists. Though her faith waivered in how much of my disease was physical, she still supported me in front of relatives, co-workers, friends, and teachers. She advocated for me in hospitals and doctors' appointments. Considering the blurriness of my diagnosis, she took a considerable leap of faith and went to incredible lengths to combat her skepticism.

However, in my family, the reality of my situation often got lost in translation. Most of my family members had different theories on why I was unwell. Sometimes these judgments were innocent. Other times, they were downright malicious. Here were some of their conclusions:

- I was doing this to myself because of my diet. ("She should be gluten free!" "She should be on Paleo." "She needs to eat more, not less!")

- I was taking too much/the wrong kind of medication. ("She obviously just needs to be on Xanax all the time." "If she would just get off all those crazy medications, I'm sure she'd be fine." "Can't they just give her something to make her normal again?" "She really needs to get prescribed something to fix that.")

- I enjoyed the daily life of a patient. ("Sure, I'd fake an illness too if it meant I got to stay home all day and never have to work a real job." "Wow, she really likes going to those doctors' appointments, doesn't she?" "I think she likes all the attention she gets in the emergency room.")

There's plenty to judge when you're a witness and not the patient. Life-long diseases test your decision-making skills and make people around you confident that they could make better choices. The people in your life will have unease about your disease. They may express this through teasing, failing to be there for you, or arguing about your treatment plan. Learning how to recognize this unease, and understanding that it is a defense technique and not about your worth as a person in need of support, is a start to building the support system that you will most definitely need.

The Fallout of Support

When you find yourself sick, your relationships will undoubtedly be tested. There comes a time when you will have no choice but to mindfully examine your friendships. Who will step up? What role will they play in making that relationship even stronger? Who will raise you up? Who will let you down and why? It is a bummer to think about, but it is common for people to let you down. Feeling powerless doesn't feel good, and your family and friends will do their best to avoid it. The most likely result is that their support for you will fall away.

How does that work? What does this fallout look like? When someone first gets severely injured in an accident, the people in their world rush to give support. Who wouldn't want to be there for a friend or family member in need, incapacitated and probably depressed about having to postpone their life for a few days or possibly weeks? The second time someone gets injured, the support system tends to rally just a little slower, providing a little less encouragement, and they may even jokingly question if that person is intentionally getting into accidents for the sympathy, the days it will leave them out of work, or a variety of other excuses.

Having a chronic illness works the same way. Let's take Joey's story as an example of how this fallout of support can happen. At twenty five years old, my older sister's boyfriend, Joey, was diagnosed with a rare form of pancreatic cancer. I remember the feeling of my stomach dropping as I listened to her breaking the news over the phone. I raced to show my support, to do my share of research, to make calls, send care packages, and be an ear for venting frustrations. I had been a patient in crisis, and I knew exactly what to do. Two weeks later, none of Joey's or my sister's friends managed to show any sign of support or comfort. My heart broke for them again. Why weren't people popping out of the woodwork to be there for them? My sister asked me on the phone, "Exactly what part of 'My boyfriend has pancreatic cancer' do they not understand?" I knew my sister had great friendships with people all over the country. Didn't they know what a crisis this was? That's when I realized that, no, they probably didn't. They probably had no idea what this could be like. They were young adults who most likely had never known someone that was their age with cancer. They didn't know if what Joey needed was support or privacy. They probably had no idea what to say, so they said nothing at all.

Sound familiar? Support is not an instinct. It doesn't come naturally to people who have never experienced that level of disaster. It doesn't mean they don't care, that they don't want to care, or that they're "bad people" for not diving head first into the water to fish you out. While some may try ineffectually (and sometimes offensively) to support you, others may completely vanish altogether. What they say about you isn't fueled by you or your disease, but rather, it is greatly influenced by how small and ineffective they feel in the face of something so large and ambiguous that they have no power to make better.

People Need Information and Experience to Effectively Show Support

In most cases, the people in your life will not be able to fully relate to what you're going through. They may not have a chronic illness. They may not have experienced being a caregiver or an emotional support for another patient in their lives. Help them to help you by communicating what it is that is happening, how you're feeling about it, and maybe even linking them to some resources explaining what your condition is and how it progresses. Most importantly, let them know that their support is key to you getting through this. A statement like that will empower them to go the extra mile, learn about your illness, and feel like they have an important role to play in your recovery.

They Need to Understand the Diagnosis. Consider sending them links to a website that might explain it more plainly. Sharing these kinds of informative articles on social media can also help friends get a clearer view of what's going on behind the scenes.

They Need to See What Has Changed. Before Joey's diagnosis, he was your average Seattle-based twenty-something. Then, he lost thirty pounds in a short amount of time, could no longer work, and had to take time off his day job. He felt pain across his back and abdomen from where the tumor was pressing on his spleen and liver. But Joey still looked like Joey. How could anyone really notice a difference in him?

They Need to Understand the Treatment. On his first day of chemo, everyone in Joey's sphere of support was on pins and needles. We'd all heard what kind of aggressive treatment he was about to receive. We knew that he would likely feel sick and nauseated, and be drugged and in pain. We were informed. There were plenty of people in Joey's life who cared for him, but how could they know how critical a day like that could be if they didn't really know much about how chemo works?

They Need to Know That They're Needed. After weeks of radio silence from friends and relatives, my sister finally allowed me to set up a donation site to help Joey afford some alternative treatment options to deal with his side effects, help cover some living costs while they took off work to navigate treatment, and make sure they had back-up funds for emergencies. I created the site and put up a detailed story of what had happened so far in his treatment and what the next steps were. Within two days we raised several thousand dollars, most of which came from their friends and family. But what came with each donation mattered most. The notes of love and support came flooding in, and with them, notes of regret for not understanding the gravity of the situation sooner.

A Diagnostic Mouthful: When They're Ready to Listen, What Do I Say?

Learning to talk to your family about your disease is one of the largest hurtles you'll encounter. Educating them about your disease can sometimes feel like trying to teach advanced trigonometry to a four-year-old. But, learning to communicate on this topic is the best way to avoid misunderstanding and to assuage their lingering feelings of powerlessness.

You must communicate with people who have their hands over their ears. When people you love don't understand what is really happening, you may find they don't stick around. I'd even recommend over-communicating with them! Write an email. Send a letter. Make a phone call. Write a status update. Spell it out with chocolate frosting. Embarrass them with a singing telegram.

What happens when you're confronted about your disease and asked to explain it and you freeze? Where do you even start? It can be kind of crazy how long you could go on about *what* your disease has done to your life without mentioning *how*. Your disease can feel like an insurmountable thing to describe on the spot. I know mine did. Let's break it down by looking at some of the major impacts your disease has on your day. Here are some questions to get you started thinking about how you would respond:

Do I wake up feeling good? Or, do I wake up feeling like I haven't slept at all?

Do I have to take multiple medications before getting a move on in the morning?

Do I need to use assistive devices or avoid parts of my normal morning routine?

Do I have to think more deliberately about how comfortable the clothes are that I'll need to wear?

Do I have to make decisions about every meal? What will give me the most energy? What could possibly throw me into a flare? What do I have in my fridge that won't make me sick?

Do I go to a job that I worry I'll lose because my employers might find me less valuable if they know about my disease?

Do I have the energy for a social life anymore?

Do I have to spend all my money on medical expenses?

You'll also want to decide how much you want others to know when it comes to the details of your condition.

Are you comfortable sharing the details on what your feeding tube or ostomy bag helps with?

Do you want them to know about what kind of medications you take, or treatments you take part in?

Do you want them to know how many doctors you see? How often you're hospitalized?

The answers to these questions will vary from person to person. Your long-distance relative who you rarely see and only talk with on the phone once a year may not need to know about the results from your last blood test, but your best friend has probably been waiting to hear back about it just as anxiously as you have. Your co-workers may need to know specifics about how your environment impacts your disease, such as keeping the thermostat at an even temperature, not being able to sit through long meetings, or having to telecommute from time to time. You may even want to alter your responses based on how much time you have to explain it, whether or not you're in a professional or social setting, or simply how open you feel that day. Whatever your decision, it helps to develop a standard elevator pitch.

How Can I Quickly Explain My Disease?

There's been far too many embarrassing moments in my life where I've had to introduce myself and then my disease in the same breath. Quickly summing up primary immune deficiency (let alone the other illnesses I've been diagnosed with) in one breath takes Olympic lungs that I just don't have.

Ever heard of something called an elevator pitch? It's a term used to describe a short statement that quickly sums up a business proposal. Getting a person to understand the intricacies of life with a rare or chronic disease in just a few short words will be useful in many life situations. An elevator pitch may end up being one of your greatest tools when it comes to advocating for your needs or accommodations. Here are some tips on perfecting your pitch quickly and accurately without getting that blank stare in return.

Ask Before You Explain. It's rare, but sometimes people have heard of your disease and don't even need to hear your spiel. Before breaking into the song and dance, preface your pitch by saying, "I have a disease called primary immune deficiency, are you familiar with it?" This statement does two things. It verifies whether someone knows what your disease already is, and it gives them the option of asking for more information if they don't. After all, nothing is weirder than an unsolicited lesson on your complicated health issues.

Don't Get Too Technical. Instead of focusing on the pathology of your disease or breaking down the genetics of it, try to focus on how the disease affects you as a person. You may want to say that because of this disease you're more susceptible to infection, which means you might have to be more cautious than the average person. You may choose to say that your body doesn't produce the natural defenses against infection, so you have medication to replace it. Or, that some days you feel completely normal and can function just like everyone else, and some days you feel like you got hit by a train.

Use Analogies or Familiarities. What can you relate your disease to that this person will understand? This can be altered for situations in which you're speaking to children, adults, and even doctors who are unfamiliar with your condition. People with Crohn's disease might say something like, "Living with Crohn's is like carrying around a ticking time bomb; one wrong bite and you could set off a painful stomach ache that can knock you out for the rest of the day or week." I've heard others describe immune disorders as, "Having a chronic illness is like being the only one casually walking through a war zone every day without any armor on, and then people are shocked and confused when you get a few bullet holes in your chest."

Mention What It Doesn't Affect. This part is one patients often forget to include. Don't forget to tell inquiring minds what you still *can* do despite your disease. Remind them that you can still work, go to school, see your friends, or go out for a few hours a day. Let them know if you can still do things like communicate online or on the phone and see your family and friends. This helps remove yourself from the pity equation and gives them an in to be included in some of these parts of your life.

Keep It Short and Shut It Down. The whole point of an elevator pitch is to avoid a long-winded (and often depressing) conversation about your disease. Keep your explanation short, concise, and to the point: "This is what I have, this is how it works, now let's go get some tacos!" A good way to bring the conversation to a screeching halt is to say something along the lines of, "It's kind of complicated, but I hope that explained some of it. You can always Google it later if you want. Wikipedia might give you a better idea of how it all goes down."

Remember that the way you discuss your disease is the way that others will interpret it. If you give a humorless, depressing description of your disease, you'll inevitably leave your audience bummed out. Don't be afraid to have fun with it. For instance, you could finish your speech by gently grasping their shoulder and saying, "...and it's highly, *highly* contagious. Just kidding!"

My Elevator Speech

When it came to developing my own elevator speech, I knew I had to find a way to describe my rare diseases in a more familiar way. I also realized that while my diseases were serious, it would create a very weird vibe if I went into the doom and gloom of how it impacted my life. I had to keep it light. It took a while, but here is the elevator speech I ultimately came up with:

I have two diseases, primary immune deficiency and dysautonomia, ever heard of them? That's okay. No one usually has! One affects my immune system. Have you ever seen that movie The Boy in the Plastic Bubble? *It's kind of like that, but not as serious and way more under control. Just give me a heads up if you have anything contagious though, okay? I also have a neurological disease that throws my autonomic system into disaster mode. Anything that should be automatic in the body—heart, sleep, temperature, and digestion—is basically running on manual via a ton of medication. The bad news is that there's not really any one specific treatment for this. The good news is that I've become extremely multi-task-oriented.*

Ready? Now it's your turn to talk! How would you explain your condition to a new person in your life? Write down some elevator speech drafts in your journal and then try them out.

Extended Family and Estranged Family

Your nuclear family is one challenge, but your extended family and your estranged family are a whole new ball game. Keeping your extended family in the loop should be done on an as needed (and as wanted) basis. Technically, if your disease is not going to affect your extended family, they don't need to understand what you're going through in-depth. If you don't prefer their help with things like getting to and from doctor's appointments or having them visit while you're in the hospital, there is no rule saying you have to say anything other than, "I'm sick, but I'm managing it."

If you have an estranged relative, maybe a parent who you no longer keep an active relationship with, I find the best way to communicate any update in your health is via email. After all, this isn't a discussion; it's a notification.

Dealing with the Accusations of a Factitious Disorder

Experiencing your loved ones turn away from you during a period of illness is heartbreaking. However, there are even worse scenarios that can occur when sharing the details of your disease. For example, one mother, Paula, recalls the horror story of her time in court fighting for treatment for her youngest child with an immune and antibody deficiency disease: "My husband's accusations that I was 'over-medicalizing' my child caused the Department of Children and Families to start an investigation on me. It was unreal." As unreal as it feels, it is ignorant to think that even court judges are above the standard response to a complicated and invisible illness. Paula continues, "The judge, in our case, said she did a little bit of searching online about my daughter's illness, and that she concluded that it was not a real disease. I was floored. I was standing there with medical documents clearly stating her diagnosis from top board certified doctors. Throughout our time in court the judge refused to look at the documents and refused to hear from my daughter's doctor as an expert witness."

This situation seems difficult to believe, but unfortunately, it's one that's happening all too frequently to families with children touched by invisible illness. The number of autoimmune and other inflammatory diseases without known cures is on the rise. Medicine is slowly catching up in recognizing that they do exist.

When a child is sick and doesn't recover in a reasonable amount of time there may be inquiries into whether or not the child is being abused, neglected, malnourished, or whether they're having behavioral issues or not. When these kinds of situations are called into question during legal proceedings it can result in loss of custody, even when a parent is trying their best to get answers. For Paula, her case was finally settled without losing custody. She was also able to find support from other parents who had been through similar traumas. Though Paula's case is extreme, it is illustrative of the common response to accuse rather than relate.

A problem Wiggins identifies as also being particularly damaging for the undiagnosed is being accused of faking their illness. "Patients suffering without diagnostic confirmation may also suffer inaccurate accusations like factitious disorder (formerly known as Munchausen)." And, family members aren't always the only ones capable of damaging accusations. Wiggins points out that even doctors can do it. "In my experience, doctors are trained to be experts and pride themselves on being good diagnosticians with the ability to provide appropriate treatment. I have witnessed countless medical professionals assure a patient with a rare diagnosis that his or her unique approach to medicine will provide a cure or solution, when in the end, the doctor was not able to affect any change. This is frustrating for both doctor and patient. When doctors can't find solutions, they respond the way many people respond to failure—blame. In this case, a doctor feeling inadequate to solve a medical problem may blame the problem on the patient or caregiver by referencing factitious disorder."

No one needs a heaping pile of blame in addition to the already burdensome life of chronic illness. In my experience, I grew up around doctors who accused me of faking or exaggerating symptoms. They sneered. They prescribed me medications I'd already tried. They told me to change my diet, exercise regimen, or sleeping schedule. They told me it was all in my head. Or, they would take one look at my chart and assure me it wasn't all in my head, but that nothing could be done. In the absence of blame and frustration, there is only one remaining response: a declaration of powerlessness and an apology because they know they won't be the one able to help you.

When it comes to dealing with doctors who believe you may be faking your symptoms, Wiggins advises: "If you are someone who has been accused of faking symptoms or factitious disorder by your doctor, stay calm and consider finding a new medical provider. Be honest with your treatment team, tell them if you have experienced this accusation and demonstrate your willingness to cooperate with diagnostic or investigative suggestions that will lead to proper diagnosis."

When someone blames you for a problem, your automatic response may be to defend yourself. Defensiveness only increases your own anxiety and feelings of self-doubt. In the instance of being blamed or accused of something untrue, instead of defending, try to problem solve in a productive manner by seeking treatment by professionals that think outside of the box and are eager to support your health and wellbeing. Though your first reaction may be feelings of anger or hopelessness, try to resist. You know your body; don't allow your observations to be denied. You may not have your answers yet, but you must keep working towards them through meticulous documentation, organization, and by not letting your emotions color your path to better health. Sometimes that means seeing a therapist to help you deal with the real impact of living with incredible medical stress. This is also helpful on another level since your primary doctor may request that your mental health be professionally evaluated.

Sharing Your Truth, Establishing Boundaries, and Finding Forgiveness

Hopefully, this chapter has provided some understanding of how and why others react the way they do to mentions of your disease. The tools learned here, like your elevator speech, will help you to share your story quickly and without awkwardness. You should now have a better idea of which people in your life you may need to take a step back from and which people you should give a chance to understand what you're going through. Finding forgiveness for those who fail to support you along the way takes time and many conversations you never thought you'd need to have with the people who are supposed to love you no matter what.

For many people, family is a tough social network to navigate, whether they live far away or intentionally distance themselves. When family members make themselves unavailable, it's good to have new faces to turn to. In the next chapter, we'll discuss how you can keep your illness from alienating you socially.

CHAPTER 4

Making New Friendships and Salvaging Old Ones

Didn't think you'd need a how-to guide on how to make friends after kindergarten, did you? Don't be embarrassed. Chronic illness can make you miss out on a lot of great things, including building those friendships and relationships that you need to stay strong and feel normal. When you're just trying to stay above water with work or school, getting your treatment settled, and trying to find your footing each time a fresh wave of symptoms hits, who has time for a social life?

The answer is that you do. Or rather, you *should* make time. Think of your social life as being as vital as any other treatment for your disease, not as a privilege for the healthy. The U. S. National Academy of Sciences conducted a study in 2016 that "found that a higher degree of social integration was associated with lower risk of physiological dysregulation in a dose-response manner in both early and later life. Conversely, lack of social connections was associated with vastly elevated risk in specific life stages" (Yang, et al. 2015). In other words: Make friends or risk spending most of your time focusing on and thus intensifying your worst symptoms. Your network gives you an outlet to forget, refocus, push through, and at the worst of times, well, they might just make you laugh.

As you move out of high school and college, or you need to resort to home schooling or telecommuting for your career, you've probably realized that it is *really* hard to make friends when there aren't that many people you get to interact with daily. Try to remember that inevitablity there will be periods in your life that you will be alone. This isn't exclusive to those with chronic illness; this is an entirely human experience that happens to everyone as they struggle to figure out who they are and with whom they feel comfortable. Don't panic. This isn't forever. Remember what we discussed in chapter one about acceptance. You aren't defeated. You aren't forgotten. Don't heap any more self-defeating thoughts on to yourself. Accept that this moment happens universally.

Just because you've been alone for a long time doesn't mean that you can't have a social recovery. There is always a time and a chance to make new friends or recover old ones. "Coming out" about my disease was like stepping out into the sun while squinting. I didn't know what was going to come at me. I worried about insults and accusations of faking or attention-seeking. But, when I finally opened my eyes and took in the world around me, I found understanding and compassion from others that I hadn't even yet learned to give to myself.

This chapter will give many examples of how to maintain old and new friendships. Ultimately, the true test of a lasting friendship is how badly both of you want it to continue despite whatever you might endure in life.

How to Maintain Friendships

Chronic illness has made me look at my friendships in a totally new way. The nature of each friendship is different. For example, I have a friend I have dinner with every few months, and we end up catching up for hours because we don't see each other often. I have a friend who works near my neighborhood and likes to come by on her lunch hour and hang out with me before she heads back to work. I have a group of friends that I gather for parties at my house, even if I haven't seen them since last year's pumpkin carving bash. I have a friend in New York who I only got to see for twenty minutes earlier this year, but being wrapped up in her arms had me feeling all the emotion and love of a twenty-year-long friendship.

Friendships change according to the seasons of your life. This would happen whether you were sick or healthy. Sometimes you might take a sabbatical from a friendship and find yourself walking back in as if nothing has happened a year later. Do your best to hang on to the good friends, the ones who make the effort to support you even when you can barely support yourself. Here are a few ways to maintain friendships, even when you find yourself unavailable.

Speak Up: Don't be afraid to tell your friends what's happening in your life. If you're having a particularly rough flare, at least give them the opportunity to be there for you by letting them know. I was surprised how many people stepped out of the woodwork when I finally started opening up about how often I was in the hospital.

Check In: Make sure there is never too long of a gap in the conversation. Keep your buddies nearby via text messages, phone calls, Facebook, etc. For me, writing a blog about my journey was my invitation for support. You don't have to write a novel about your disease, but consider writing a Facebook status and letting others know when you've checked into the ER or have been admitted to the hospital.

Make the Plans: Don't leave it up to your friends to set a date. Take control by making low-key, realistic plans for your energy level. Maybe go for a quiet night out at a restaurant whose menu you know you can eat from. You can even invite friends over to watch a new release on Netflix or to create a new recipe together.

Why Are You Not Making Friends?

There are some very universal reasons that chronic illness patients struggle with making friends. We struggle with shame and worthiness. You may think, *Who would want to be friends with someone who cancels plans, spends long periods of time in the hospital, and is constantly in some amount of discomfort or pain?*

Shame is a natural reaction to having an illness. For many people, shame sneaks in without a name or a face and completely alters your perception of yourself. It is the most hazardous factor in preventing you from connecting with other people. Shame makes you hide things and pretend things are fine when they're extremely painful. Not only are social situations difficult to get through, it becomes harder and harder to believe that being with other people can be enjoyable. How lonely! When I think about failures in friend-making when I was younger, I know it goes a lot deeper than not sharing the same interests. You might lack the confidence to share yourself with others when you don't know how or when to "reveal" your disease.

Before I knew what my disease was, I was hiding it. Keeping my symptoms quiet and concealed around other people was my marching order. Do you ever feel like that's been your experience? The truth is that my disease made me feel very different from other people. I always had this chip on my shoulder and felt like I could never take things to the next level. I couldn't get close to people because I felt that eventually I would flare up and let them down. It took me many years to find the strength to even try to be someone's friend. It took even more time to learn that unlike for other people, keeping and strengthening those friendships was going to take effort and commitment. But, having those lonely stretches without a social life gave me more strength to pursue and appreciate my friendships when I finally did have the opportunity to connect with people.

Making and breaking plans is a common theme for people with chronic illness. It doesn't change much from being a sickly ten-year-old to a sickly twenty-four-year-old. Finding the right restaurants to eat at, deciding on activities that won't require much activity, and having to cancel last minute for things you can't really control makes it tricky to maintain close friendships. Uneasiness with your disease is extremely obvious to others. When you start to get comfortable about your condition, you'll put others at ease as well and it will be easier to make friends and maintain those relationships.

How to Start Making Friends

If you've been off the social stratosphere for way too long, to the point where you're having intense conversations with your dog or crying into your birthday cake while your mom watches on, it's okay, it happens.

Getting back in the saddle after a long flare-up can feel like you are attempting to meaningfully converse in another language when you only know how to say, "where is the bathroom?" You may have completely lost confidence in yourself and your ability to make friends and that's expected. Here are some reminders and ideas of ways to connect with people.

1. **Draw on Your Current Contacts:** Check in to see how old friends are doing. Use your social networks to send messages and see if they might want to get coffee soon. Remember who you used to hang out

with in healthier times and reconnect. Ask how their lives have changed since you last spoke.

2. **Be Kind:** Seems obvious, right? Make a conscious effort to be kind. Compliment a stranger. Make a comment to a classmate or coworker about their presentation during a meeting. Congratulate another mom at the park for keeping her cool when her kid went all "*Exorcist* style" on the monkey bars for not being allowed to have candy. Kindness invites kindness, so don't be afraid to notice someone's better qualities.

3. **Reach Out:** During my first year of high school, I spent the first week or two having lunch by myself. I had homeschooled the year before and now finding myself in a crowd of other teenagers felt really jarring. Then, out of the clear blue, a girl tapped me on the shoulder and asked me to come and sit with her and her friends. She did it with such confidence and nonchalance. Why after all these months had I not asked another person if I could sit with them? Reach out. Just ask. You very well may be the only person excluding yourself from a social life.

4. **Get Their Contact Info:** Once you've made a connection with someone, make sure you ask for their phone number and let them know you'll text them soon to hang out.

5. **Don't Fear Spontaneity:** If your symptoms are mostly under control for the day, and a conversation results in an invitation to hang out, go for it! Seize the moment to socialize as often as your body allows you to.

Where Can You Meet People?

Patients with chronic illness do not have a monopoly on loneliness. Everyone goes through periods of time where they outgrow old friends before finding new ones. It's difficult, especially in your adult years, to effortlessly slide into a group of people who you can connect with. But there are places to make friends. I've provided some ideas below to get you started.

Meet Friends Online

One of the hardest questions is "Where are all the people?" They weren't in my living room. They weren't at my doctor's office. My first foray into finding new friendships came from the internet and connecting with others who had a chronic illness. The positive aspect of this was that I no longer had to hold back and hide the symptoms of my disease. I could share my challenges at leisure. The downside was that often, besides our diseases, we really had nothing else in common. Sometimes these friendships tended to turn into merely sounding boards for complaints about our diseases.

In the earlier days of my diagnosis, I would do online searches of the main organizations for my disease and set up an account to get in their chat rooms or forums. Later, I discovered a huge and ever-expanding series of Facebook groups for people with chronic illnesses. Many communities had 5,000 members or more who were all reading and responding to posts in real time. The benefit of this was checking to see if things were normal. People would pop in and ask questions like, "Is it normal for my heart to be racing this fast?" In a few seconds, there would be fifty responses from other patients who had been there before.

Sometimes I'd get brave and ask to go to lunch with someone from an online group who lived nearby me. These lunch dates were very reaffirming since we shared similar daily realties. I started to wonder though if I would only be able to connect with people with chronic illness. How would someone who wasn't ill know how to be a friend to someone as complicated as me?

As we discuss different kinds of support later in the book, you'll see the incredible value of finding friends in similar situations, but certainly they were not the end-all, be-all to my social needs. In the meantime, virtual friends can provide streaming support on those quiet nights at home.

Make Friends at School and Work

School and work may be the easiest venue for finding new friends. You're already with people your own age, who at least have an education or career in common with you. There's plenty of opportunity to talk at lunch, before classes and meetings, and during breaks. Even at the height of my disease, during my last year in college, I managed to make a very fragile friendship with a girl who sat behind me in class. Once or twice we tested each other with flashcards in the cafeteria before tests. Because I had to leave school, I thought I had lost a potential friendship. Months went by, and then by happenstance she appeared at a house party my boyfriend had dragged me to and we were able to reconnect.

That's the thing about friendships. They don't always start with a flash and a bang. Sometimes they come in the form of acquaintances you see every now and then and grow to become strong friendships. Be open to all opportunities by being kind and open with everyone you interact with. You have nothing to be ashamed of by putting yourself out there. Co-workers might not immediately seem to have the same after-work social life as you, but give yourself time to get to know them.

When You Make a Connection

There may be no better feeling in the world than the one you get sitting across from someone who you fully connect with. It's like taking off too-tight sneakers after a long walk. There is an incredible relief and appreciation for the moment. You weren't sure if the opportunity to connect would ever actually come again and it did! You broke through! Despite the wall that your disease can build around you, you found a window, popped your head out, and waved to someone on the other side. Things are looking up. Now that you have made a connection, there are a few things to be mindful of.

Make Plans You Can Keep

After the friendly flirting and Netflix queue comparison, you've finally landed a friend-date! And, since you likely just met this person, you probably haven't told them all the details of your disease. The thought of making plans seems like an insurmountable challenge because you want to appear normal and do normal-activity-level things for someone your age, eat normal every-day food like someone your age, and discuss normal age-appropriate life experiences, but you don't quite fit into any of those bubbles.

Different diseases present different challenges to hanging out. It's not something the healthy have to think about. But you do, so let's knock some things out of the equation right now.

Eating spicy foods when it upsets your stomach? Don't do it just because everyone else wants to order the chili! Getting in line for the new rollercoaster when your worst symptom is vertigo? Don't do it. Intense physical exercise like endurance hiking or fast-paced aerobic classes? Find another activity.

If it makes you feel any better, I've learned all this from trying to pretend that I'm on the same peak physical level as my friends.

I nearly dislocated my ankle (twice) while ice skating, went to see an IMAX movie in the middle of a migraine flare, and even had something as simple as a slice of pizza ruin a perfectly good evening.

You don't have to cater to the wants and whims of your disease, but throwing caution to the wind in your effort to feel like one of the guys or girls will end badly. Believe me. Aim for a mid-week hangout with close friends by inviting them over for foods that require low-impact prep (i.e., frozen finger foods, chips, and salsa) and drinks. Invest in some board games or suggest an on-demand Bravo marathon. This sort of night gives you a chance to control the activity level. If you can aim for a smaller, less strenuous night out, you'll have more energy to focus on making a lasting connection with your friends.

Inevitably, even the most clever and capable of us will make a colossal social snafu. Don't be afraid to brush aside the compulsion to be just like everyone else. Maybe you can't enter the pie-eating contest, but there's something for everyone at the county fair.

Get Over Your Guilt

There was no question about it. If I was going to have a normal social life, I needed a major shift in attitude. The first thing that had to stop was the guilt. It was eating me up inside every time I had to cancel plans. At some point, I swore off making plans completely. After that lonely period, I made a resolution to do the opposite. I decided to make plans at every opportunity offered to me, even when I wasn't hundred percent sure I'd be able to follow through with them.

If living with a chronic, progressive disease taught me anything at all, it was that life is too short to feel bad about things you can't change. Nobody wants to be that asshole who backs out at the last minute, but sometimes it's the only way to stay connected with friends when a good deal of your life is tests, doctors, hospitals, and nights on the bathroom floor. It also became obvious that people were reflecting my attitude back at me. If I felt horrible about making and breaking plans and made a huge show of apologizing and berating myself, they felt equally horrible. If I brushed it off and said we'd try again, they mirrored my fluidity.

These days I have a group of girlfriends who I hang out with regularly. At this point they already know my whole story and then some. They've been very understanding and take it in stride when I'm not able to make it out every time we make plans. It would have sounded crazy to me just two years ago if someone had told me I'd have a lot of friends and I'd hang out with them enough to maintain those friendships.

You may think you're the only one who is tired because you have a chronic illness, but even "normal" people with "realistic" amounts of energy get tired during the week. I used to beat myself up about not always being able to go out with friends, until I realized that their relationships, landlord issues, and work drama were pretty fatigue-inducing as well. Don't let your fatigue isolate you.

How to Reveal Your Disease

In my mind, I basically have a secret identity. When I meet new people, I try to stay cool and act normal, but underneath my dress and cardigan there lies a ridiculously good-looking body wrapped up in a Holter monitor and a hospital gown. When getting to know the new people in your life, it's important to remember not to take off your dress and cardigan at the dinner table. Even if you do feel antsy about letting your secret identity be known immediately, breaking the news about the impact of your disease on your life is a delicate process. It takes thought, precision, and almost no partial-nudity. This would be a great time to use your elevator pitch. Be quick, clear, and upbeat. Still not sure what to say? Check out these five tips for the big reveal.

Reveal That You Deal with an Illness on a Need-to-Know Basis: Before revealing your situation to them, ask yourself: Is the topic of my disease bound to come up between us eventually? Do I have any obvious signs of this disease that they might start to build their own (and possibly incorrect) assumptions about? Will this person be affected by how this disease affects me? Consider whether you'll be making plans with them or working side-by-side on projects at work. If you feel your symptoms may interfere at some point, it's okay to give them a heads up.

Lastly, ask yourself: Do they care? You don't need a pat on the back and someone to call you their personal hero every time you say, "I have a serious illness." But, if someone in your life has already expressed prejudice against someone with disabilities or seems to otherwise be incredibly tactless, it might just be better to let him figure it out (or not) on his own.

Don't Overshare: Sometimes we get so used to having to explain our disease, we accidently overshare. We don't want to have our listener internally screaming—"*way* too much information!" Save it for your friends in med school who are no longer shocked by any function of the human body.

Be the Reaction You Want to Have: People are going to follow your lead when it comes to the state of your disease. If you're frustrated about it, they will be frustrated about it. If you're sad about it, they'll be sad about it. If you're cool about it, they'll be cool about it. People can sense your uneasiness about your condition. If you haven't come to terms with it yet and are still in a phase of mourning your old life, you may not be ready to reveal your experiences and open yourself up to possible judgment. You've got to love yourself with or without the disease if you're going to expect someone new in your life to do the same.

Make it Common Knowledge: What's easier than having to explain to everyone you know that you have a chronic illness? Having the internet do it! Don't be *that* guy who tweets about his medications all day long, but try posting on your social network periodically about how you're coping with your disease. This can help break the ice when you see old friends in person and could lower the shock factor with new acquaintances.

The Friend Who Gets It

If your friendships have been superficial or fleeting, just remember that true friendships do exist. They are built and maintained with effort and patience, and you will find yourself in the right ones. I've had my fair share of blank social calendars, but I've had my lucky days too. Once upon a time I had this best friend, Nikki, who got me on a real, deep personal level. Like on the kind of level where I might say in the middle of watching a movie, "I'm going to need to leave the movie now so I can go home and lay on my bathroom floor and die." And, then she would just nod, grab her purse, and say, "Let's go."

I thought this was because she too had an invisible chronic illness that she already knew by name and had already dealt with the first few years of emotional hurdles. While she was by no means cured when I met her, she still made plans, went places, and had a wild personality that her illness just couldn't dampen. Although she was often bedridden and on the other side of the bathroom door, she always had friends nearby. The more I watched her deal with her problems, the more I wanted to be just like her. But what was it that made her so *Nikki*? It was an equation that would take many terrible episodes of her disease to witness.

It wasn't that she didn't *feel* her disease or acknowledge that it was there. She just didn't hate herself for it. She didn't blame herself. For most of my life, my disease was this intangible monster that I was somehow supposed to keep locked in the closet while it howled and rattled the doors. Things like that never disappear. Shame was all it really needed to grow and I was feeding it every day. Nikki knew no fear and no blame.

You know what happens to the sick, shamed monster you keep in your closet? One day it knocks the door right off the hinges, takes a rattling breath, and tumbles out. This is one of the many reasons why it is so special if you are lucky enough to have friends who will help you through the stages of accepting your disease. It's even better if you're able to find friends who have the same struggles as you and can guide you and show you that life with chronic illness doesn't have to be a lonely road. In my experience, these friendships tend to be built on total shamelessness. In this friendship, I stopped lying, not just to another person, but to myself, and that changed everything.

Good friendships, whatever they look like, can help you in your journey to accept your circumstances and even buffer shame. They can be a buoy of support in times of chaos and a network to help you reach others. They can give you a sense of normalcy and lightheartedness even when you feel unstable. Don't ever close yourself off to friendships at any stage of your illness. While at some points you'll have do it alone, people need people to walk through the shadows with. Don't ever stop looking for a friend. There is somebody out there who needs you as a friend. My mom always says, "If you need a friend, be a friend."

CHAPTER 5

Dating and Relationships

If you thought accepting your situation, feeling positive about yourself, communicating with relatives, and making friends was hard, dating and relationships can be even more challenging. Starting relationships with people you intend to share your body with, in all its unexpected malfunctions, can be difficult to wrap your head around. It can be unnerving to create an online dating profile that spells out your inaccessibility, overbearing symptoms, and vulnerabilities.

In this chapter, we're going to explore dating, long-term relationships, sex, and partners as caregivers. Sex and relationships are not a privilege only for the healthy. People with extreme, advanced diseases still find and celebrate love. All of us are deserving of intimacy and worthy of profound love. Finding a partner who can be there to care of you, comfort you, and remind you of the positive things in life is a risk worth taking. With communication and patience, sex and love can play a crucial part in expanding your quality of life.

Dating with an Illness

Getting out in the dating world and having multiple relationships may be the only way for you to meet your match. While you may be kissing a lot of frogs, you can still protect yourself from the risk of disease and rejection by being open and honest about your disease from the get-go. Dating is a great opportunity to use your handy elevator speech. It will also help you gauge whether your potential new partner can tango with you and all your quirks. It's better to know this sooner rather than later, so that you don't find yourself sitting in a bathroom stall during your third date and trying to add an extra layer of cover-up to your surgical scars.

Ten Helpful Guidelines for Dating with an Illness

1. **Use Technology to Bypass First Date Anxiety:** Whether you're creating a profile on a dating site, or you're chatting up someone on Facebook, make sure to drop the bomb before the first date. If they don't want to go out with you after learning you have a chronic illness, then that's that. As my momma says: *next!* Breaking the news online or even over the phone early on allows your potential date to react in privacy. Since their first reaction may be confusion, giving them their own time to process the information protects them and you. You won't have to witness them stumbling to come up with a supportive, appropriate, and charming response. It allows them the ability to untangle this information before you meet for your first date, so that when you do meet in person, they'll have let it settle in their mind a bit and will be able to ask you some appropriate questions about how your disease affects your life.

2. **Don't Be a Victim:** As mentioned in the previous chapter, it's all about attitude. People are going to follow your lead when it comes to the state of your disease.

People can sense your uneasiness about your disease. If you haven't come to terms with it yet and are still in a phase of mourning your old life, you probably aren't ready to date anyway, and that's okay. Give yourself time and space. You've got to love yourself first if you're going to expect someone new in your life to do the same. Lead by example and don't walk around with a chip on your shoulder that you leave in plain view. I'm not saying you need to hug your fibromyalgia lovingly in your arms every night, but you at least need to be able to get through a flare in public without openly weeping.

3. **Highlight Your Best Assets:** You're going to be as self-conscious as any other person is on a first date, so remember to play up your best assets. Remember to take a good look in the mirror! Maybe you've packed on a few prednisone pounds? If so, it's a great time to pull out that tight skirt to show that you no longer have a flat butt. Maybe you've got circles under your eyes? Then you might want to show your date just how sexy you can look in sunglasses.

4. **Don't Give TMI:** The details of your sensitive stomach. The current color of your snot. Your barely-healed laparoscopy scars. Save it for the honeymoon, kids. While you may think your relationship warrants such vulnerability on the second date, you may want to give your love a more extended period of time to bloom before describing some more of the graphic details of your disease. (Though if you must, euphemisms or simply, "I'm not feeling well, believe me you don't want to know," should be enough.)

5. **Don't Lay Down the Law:** Yes, you need someone who won't play games. You need someone who is going to be

there for you *all* the time. You need someone reliable. You need someone understanding. But, slamming your fist down on the table every time you decree a new amendment on how you will be treated as a partner is not going to win you any suitors. If you're currently dating, try to keep an open mind about your expectations. You can't tell on a first date whether they'll be able to live up to your expectations.

Take a step back. Remember that relationships are a two-way street and you've got to be willing to put out just as much as you need to take in. So why not start off this date making a mental list of how you're going to improve *their* life? Partners of those with chronic illnesses are probably the closest things to super heroes. They put up with it all and know they won't ever get as much physical effort in return.

But that doesn't mean you can't put in effort elsewhere. There are millions of things you can do for your partner, like helping them have better relationships with their family and friends, teaching them about having career goals, handling money, and being a solid parenting partner or emotional caregiver. You're not the only one with problems, so start looking for places where you can apply yourself as the solution.

6. **Don't Be a Hero:** You may have times where you'll think, "It's just a little blood...from my eyeballs. I'm good, let's eat." Rock climbing? Extreme roller coaster riding? Hot-dog-eating contests? These might not be the best first date activities for you if you have a chronic illness. Pretty much anything on the list in the previous chapter that you wouldn't do with friends, you may also want to cross off the list for a date. Don't pretend like

you're cool, and then duck into the restroom for a moment to pass out in peace. No good will come of this.

7. **Remember to Laugh About It:** Having a sense of humor when it comes to the wild adventures and unplanned mishaps that occur in daily life with a chronic illness is imperative to successfully coping with stress. When I was younger, and had frequent emergency room visits, my mother would always spend our time in the waiting room and exam room cracking jokes and coming up with creative but harmless ways to prank the doctors. She made sure that I laughed more than I cried. You do have the choice to make every situation a misery or a pleasure. When you constantly find yourself in pain or frustration, a sense of humor is one of the best ways to bolster your spirit and keep a positive attitude.

8. **Don't Be Afraid of Rejection:** If you think you won't need to be brave after the first date, you're wrong. Relationships require all kinds of bravery. From braving that first kiss to braving the first argument. So be brave and remember if someone doesn't want to be with you, there will be someone else. It's better to be happy searching for the right one than miserable with the wrong one.

9. **Learn to Adapt and Be Okay with It:** Are you going to bail sometimes? Yes. Will you spend three hours on your hair then realize you need a nap? Probably. Is the world going to end? No. Sometimes you'll want to do something with your significant other and it just won't work out because your body is fighting back. Sure, the first few times it's okay to be frustrated and embarrassed, fumble over your apologies, and stress out that they'll be upset. As my husband, R.J., always says,

"we'll adapt." Plans change. Even if it might mess with your emotions and make for a less-than-great day, it doesn't have to make for a less-than-great relationship. Life happens. You're still allowed to love and be loved.

10. **Don't Forget That You Can Be Loved:** You must always know it. Think it. Act with it in your consciousness as you propel yourself into the life of another person. You're not just a person who is chronically ill. You are a person, and you happen to also be chronically ill. Don't let your disease define your personality. You are so much more than an illness. When you stop thinking of yourself in that box, others will too. Your illness will limit a lot of things in your life, but it doesn't make you any less able to be loved. At the end of the day, dating exists to accomplish two goals: to find someone you like and to have fun. If you're not doing either, you're doing it wrong.

Trusting Someone with Your Body

I could not have fathomed the kind of anxiety I would get over French kissing someone I'd only known for six hours. It's not so sexy when, instead of keeping track of where his hands are, you're too busy contemplating whether he's recently been with someone who might have had the flu, or worse, mono. Is he the kind of guy who takes his full course of antibiotics when he gets strep throat? And all that's long before you start contemplating the mileage of his junk. It's definitely awkward when in the middle of a steamy embrace you have to whisper, "Are you excited to touch me or are you running a fever? Because if it is a fever, you've got to pack it up." For those with compromised immune systems, you'll probably have to consider the following questions before getting intimate with someone.

- How much do you trust your partner?

- Do you trust them enough to tell them the secrets you have about the strength of your body?

- Do you trust them enough to realize that their health inevitably will affect your health?

- Do you trust them to not share their body with someone else whose diseases could potentially come back to you?

I know it's kind of a 1950s view on intimacy, but in a world of so much viable birth control it can be too easy to discard the kind of options that protect you from venereal diseases. You are your body's only advocate, so don't wait on your partner to offer up information that they might not think is relevant, especially if they don't know your health status. You need to ask: Are you sick? Do you have anything communicable, even if it's not affecting your junk? If they say yes, slow down and try to prioritize what is more important: the risk of developing an infection or catching a virus, or the need to connect?

I will be perfectly honest, the need to connect physically with someone often outweighs the consequences of catching a cold. (A *cold*, not a disease.) And that's okay. You're allowed to choose pleasure over the discomfort of minor illness. However, you should consider the reality that whatever happens may have a much larger effect on you than it has on your partner's life. It could disrupt your ability to go to school or work, or even lead to a greater health crisis. The choice is yours, but you have the right to make an informed choice.

Handling the Early Stages of Romance

So how do you broach the subject of "healthy" boundaries to a date, random hook-up, or friend with benefits? In a word: honesty. What are you going to do, put yourself in mortal peril (or whatever) just to get some? Totally not judging, we've all done it. But just so we don't make it a habit, let's talk about how to break the ice when it comes to sharing your concerns. Some examples of things you could say:

- "So, fun fact: I'm immune deficient and if you're sick, we could reschedule. I'm feeling really good with you right now, but you're going to kill me. Well, maybe not kill me, but definitely knock me down for a while if that's not a bottle of cough syrup in your pants."

- "Look, the fact is that because of my fatigue I have to take naps more often than most people, which means there's a good chance we'll end up in bed together."

- "Not that I don't think it's really cool that you can walk up a hill very fast, but I don't think I'm really up to hiking on our date. Maybe we could watch a movie about hiking. I heard *127 Hours* is a good one."

You're going to be a lot more comfortable and a lot better off in the long term by just communicating. I know there's something romantic in the mystery of learning about each other, but this isn't the kind of thing you'll want to spring on someone three months into a relationship. Is it even realistic to think you could hide this for three months?

You might be worried that once you communicate about your illness, they'll be turned off, or think it's weird or TMI. If that's the case, then they kind of suck, don't they? Do you really want to be in a relationship with someone who is unsupportive about something like this right off the bat? The possibility of being rejected for our illnesses is a wound that runs deep. After being rejected by family or friends and humiliated by doctors or employers, the very idea of revealing something so personal in such a personal situation can be daunting and extremely unappealing. Let's talk about a few ways we can push through this uneasiness and open a real dialogue about how disease is handled in functional relationships.

Be Open and Accept the Unexpected Response

When you've accepted your disease, you can come at these confrontations with a new kind of confidence. You are not to be ashamed of the extra burden you carry with you every day. Your ability to even be in a dating situation where you get to a point of revealing your disease is a triumph. Be proud of your strength to come clean on the subject and expect your partner to show many responses. This includes curiosity, which is a completely normal reaction and one that they have a right to satisfy by asking questions. The second might be concern. Is this pity for you or worry for themselves about having to cope with this new element of the relationship? Maybe even genuine anguish that you need to deal with these symptoms? All normal. All part of that important discussion you'll have to have to lay the groundwork for your relationship.

If you cannot lay this foundation of understanding and support, then you are setting yourself up for a relationship full of resentment, doubt, and low self-respect. You deserve a partner who is "in it" with you, and your partner deserves the chance to fully "choose" to be in this relationships with all the facts. Here are some takeaways to help make sure that you and your partner make fully informed decisions about your relationship together.

Going Long-Term. Familiarity, in the world of chronic illness, might not actually breed contempt, especially when it comes to relationships. There are a lot of pros to being in a committed, long-term relationship when you're already dealing with the tumultuous unpredictability of your body.

Having an Informed, Educated Partner. Being in a long-term relationship means the initial bandage of explaining your illness is over quickly. Though it may take your partner some time to truly understand the impact of your disease on your life, they're at least aware it exists and you may feel no need to hide it.

Lowered Risk for Disease. Long-term relationships, especially when monogamous, provide a less stressful atmosphere around transmitting disease. If your partner is only having sex with you, you may not have to do as many health checks and have as many uncomfortable conversations before intimacy.

Comfort and Understanding in Times of Distress. While dating may be a sprint, a long-term relationship is a marathon. If you don't show up to a first date, it sets a bad impression. However, if you've been dating your partner for a long period of time and have to cancel plans, it's more likely that you'll feel less guilty knowing there will be more opportunities to be with each other.

Caretaking. Ultimately, your partner may become your caretaker. You'll have to decide just how far you'd like to extend that part of your relationship, but having a long-term partner can be a substantial help to you during bad days when you need a little extra help.

Boundaries and Caregiving

My mother always said to me, "My proudest accomplishment is getting all that long-term insurance so that you'll never have to wipe my ass when I'm senile." I'm sure this is not actually her proudest accomplishment, but it is a giant sigh of relief in the context of what our lives will look like when my mother grows old and needs that kind of help. The thought of my husband ever having to do any kind of general hygienic task beyond helping me brush my teeth is a little mortifying. I've set a boundary there and explained that if it were to get to that point I would want outside help. Or if the situation is perhaps serious but temporary, I would prefer to be hospitalized where nurses could help me in a more controlled environment. This isn't about hiding things from your partner, or about being petty about them seeing you at your worst; it's about your right to preserve your dignity and set boundaries as far as caregiving. The best way to do this may be to decide ahead of time.

So how do you know when you've reached your limit as far as what you feel comfortable letting your caregiver do? Oh, you'll feel it. Deciding ahead of time is the way to go. Consider things like: Do you care if they see you naked? Do you care if they assist you with going to the bathroom? Do you care if they assist you with bathing? Would you be mortified if they had to give you an enema? For many chronic illness patients, they've been so vigorously put through the ringer, most of these things don't faze them when a nurse does it. You just need to ask yourself: Do I want to be seen in all my inglorious glory by the same person I'm going to want to have sex with as soon as I get better?

Your partner really needs to have a say in this too! After all, this may not have been in the contract they signed at the start of your relationship. Not all partners have the desire to be caregivers. Not all of them have the capacity to be one. However, if they are going to give it a shot, you need to make the situation as comfortable for them as you're attempting to make it for yourself.

What Does Your Partner Have the Right to Expect from You?

1. **Honesty:** Your partner has the right to know when their night might be interrupted by an ER visit. If you don't tell them how badly you're feeling, how will they prepare themselves?

2. **Contributions:** Anyone can contribute. Be a thoughtful sounding board to their problems or help motivate them towards a goal.

3. **A Chance to React:** They should be able to react to every new and frustrating situation. You may have been prepared for the possibility that your disease might progress. You might need new assistive devices, surgeries (minor and life-threatening), or have reactions to your medications that alter your personality. Your partner, however, may not understand the gravity of a progressive illness and might need time and help to process life-altering changes in your health.

4. **This Isn't a Competition:** Just because you have a chronic disease doesn't mean your partner can't have a worse day than you. You still need to be a member of the team.

5. **A Break:** It takes a village, as mentioned multiple times in this book, to care for someone with a chronic illness. Make sure your partner has a night off occasionally.

6. **Adventure and Opportunity:** You may not always be able to go to the midnight showing of a movie, take a flight to Japan, or go on an airboat ride, but you can't begrudge your partner the opportunity to do these things alone or with family or friends.

Developing a Strong Bond

Being in a relationship with someone with chronic illness requires an understanding of what kind of sacrifices and precautions we need to take to maintain our health. We've discussed the perils of dating, the pros of long-term relationships, and the unexpected intimacies that come with caregiving. At the various natural stages of a relationship, more is asked of people with chronic illness. There is a greater vulnerability, a deeper sense of trust, a higher set of expectations, and an even greater possibility of rejection. When a bond is formed despite all these barricades, it is extraordinarily strong.

My husband has woven himself into the fabric of my life. He doesn't just provide a stable thread to keep the tapestry together, but bends with the motions of change. Whatever we face—unexpected surgeries to unexpected hospital bills—we continue to communicate, vent, push each other forward, and understand that neither of us will always say or do the perfect thing. He remembers that my disease is not a journey I can take on my own, and in turn I keep in mind that he can't be responsible as the sole pillar of support for all my body's extracurricular chaos.

How does this work? While at the start of our relationship I may have tried my best to hide some of my less flattering flare-ups, over time I realized that I could not keep up the act. More importantly, he didn't want me to. Give your partner the chance to support you. If they are anything like my husband, who is incredibly well-meaning but also incredibly unsure most of the time of what to do with me, walk them through it. Take their hand. Recognize that no one is hardwired with the ability to read your mind. Explain what you're experiencing, what they can do to help, and have patience as they learn about the patterns of your disease. Most of the time there will be nothing that they can do to help but to simply *be there*, riding the wave with you as you navigate through the worst of your pain or discomfort.

CHAPTER 6

Creating a Support System

You may hear the word "caretaker" and think of a nurse in scrubs changing out an IV bag or even the main person in your family who most assists you when you're at your physical worst. However, creating a support system needs to be more than just that *one* person or the list of specialists you see to treat your disease. A support system for a chronic illness patient needs to extend beyond care for physical ailments; it should also include social, emotional, and even spiritual care.

As strong as my close-knit support system is, I have created an even bigger support network to catch me when I fall. When your family, friends, and partners need a break from caregiving, you'll need other resources to turn to. Early on, before I had accepted the idea that I had a chronic illness, I hadn't really considered the possibility that I might need support. With all the humiliation I was experiencing because of my symptoms, I wondered if I even deserved support from anyone outside my immediate circle. After all, my problems weren't so serious, were they?

I was alone a lot: on the floor, on the toilet, or waiting in the exam room. I felt alone when I went on Hospital Homebound (HH) in high school and when I started taking online classes for college. I got used to being alone in the worst parts of my illness. What did I need to burden others with it for? What exactly could they do anyway? Hold my left hand while my right one knocked back my morning medications? But I needed support; it was obvious.

Having supportive friends, family, work, and school environments all serve a vital purpose. However, you'll want to remember that there is an entire other group to help support you through your hard times: your fellow patients. At some stages in your chronic illness you'll need to vent, and you'll need to have people sympathize. When you hit a wall or want to give up, you'll need people who will pull you back up and get in your face about moving forward. You'll need people to help you keep track of progress and remind you just how far you've really come.

You'll also feel the need to help others during these same experiences. Helping others to overcome their challenges keeps your skills fresh, helps you to acknowledge your accomplishments, and gives your struggle a sense of purpose.

What Kind of Support Will You Need?

Support is not optional, but you do have options on how you can obtain it. Your reach can go further than just your close family and friends. There are many infrastructures of support that you may not realize are available to you and created for patients just like you in mind. Below is a list of different kinds of support you may need.

Emotional Support

According to the National Institutes of Health, patients with chronic medical illnesses have been found to have higher rates of depression and anxiety. So, how do you go about obtaining emotional support when you feel depressed or are experiencing anxiety? How do you best resolve your emotional breakdowns? Start by thinking of that one person who you immediately dial as soon as you step out of the doctor's office with bad news. It's good to have this one friend or family member to rely on for support as your first line of defense, but they can't do it alone. You might want to consider different kinds of talk therapies, such as speaking with a psychologist or clergy member. If you don't feel like sharing the details of your situation with close friends or even just "in-person" with anyone, you can also use the internet to find patient communities to vent in and ask for guidance.

Informational Support

When you're first diagnosed with a disease, you're going to experience a few moments of panic thinking about how this disease will affect you down the road. Will it get worse? Will you still be mobile or will you require assistive devices? Will you be able to have kids or live independently? How bad will things really be?

Being in touch with those patients who share your condition but have a few more years of experience than you can be hugely beneficial. You'll be able to get a better footing on your future and adjust your habits accordingly. Learning how other patients handled their disease and what choices they made in their lives to ensure a better quality of life can help you plan, cope with reality, and begin adjusting your mind-set about the challenges ahead. For me, quickly getting online after my first diagnosis and searching for patient stories became an invaluable pasttime. I also visited the pharmaceutical website of the medication I was taking, which connected me to various patient communities.

Medical Support

As we'll explore throughout the book, particularly in chapter 9, getting effective medical support is key to successful treatment in chronic illness patients. There are other medical support options you may want to consider as well, such as home health care, rehabilitation facilities and programs, aid devices, and furniture that help in assisting with everyday movements.

For me, there have been times that my blood pressure was so out of control that I had to use a wheelchair to get around without fainting. I've also received a handicap parking pass to help me get to bathrooms more quickly when needed, and to help not exacerbate fatigue and chronic pain with long walks across hot parking lots. In the past, I've had home health nurses who've helped me to access my port, set up my IVs, care for wounds, and even just keep an eye on me when I'm on heavy doses of medications after surgeries or bad flares and I have no one else around.

Creating an Informed Support System

Once you've developed your social and medical support systems, it's time to create a system of relevant information to help you stay an informed, proactive patient. You'll want to find your disease community online, in-person, and through other experienced patients. You'll need these communities to get feedback, share advice, and find common goals within your plan of treatment.

Option 1: Finding Your Online Community

You have questions—good ones, stupid ones, rude ones—but probably many that you don't feel like asking your doctor or friends. Online communities provide that anonymity you need while giving other patients the anonymity they need to give honest answers.

Twenty minutes into my first IVIG treatment in the hospital, I whipped out my laptop and started researching. At first, I just wanted to know how I would feel during and after my first infusion. But then I realized that PrimaryImmune.org had entire forums and chatrooms for teens discussing their diagnosis. I quickly skimmed through the website and started to introduce myself. Sitting in that cold recliner, watching the gel-like liquid drip from my IV, I suddenly started to feel my dread melting away. I chatted with five other patients in the middle of getting their infusions that afternoon. They were all excitedly giving me tips and answering my questions.

Since then, I've discovered active online communities on social media sites, chatrooms, message boards, and health sites for even the rarest diseases. Through my work at Global Genes, I've seen patients connect through shared stories and meet-up events and have witnessed online organizations grow awareness, raise funds, and make change—all online! Not sure where to start? GlobalGenes.org has a full list of rare and genetic disease organizations, and TheMighty.com has a surplus of patient stories on different conditions. Searching through the groups section on Facebook for your disease will usually bring up a few different pages to post on.

What Makes a Good Online Support Group?

- Topics that are focused

- A non-hostile community with moderators who can help limit negative interactions and spam

- Groups that label conversations separately, so there's a place to vent, a place to ask questions, and a place to get patient experiences on different doctors, hospitals, and treatments

- A larger overall organization that offers online support to help provide educational, financial, or other resources

Option 2: In-Person Support Groups

Due to vertigo, I couldn't drive far. This meant that even when my health was at its worst, finding face-to-face support was difficult. For a long time, I struggled with the idea that I might never know someone who was going through what I was going through. But, after about a year after my diagnosis, with the help of my doctor, I organized a support group.

My doctor and I took several weeks to promote our group. We posted in all the online communities, sent out memos to all the chronic illness foundations, and distributed a press release to local media outlets. We then put together a PowerPoint presentation that outlined the basic symptoms of postural orthostatic tachycardia syndrome (POTS). We reserved a conference room in the hospital's learning center for 7:30 p.m. on a weeknight. We spread out the chairs, loaded up a table with sports drinks and pretzels, and waited...and waited. My mom was the first to come, excited to potentially meet other mothers whose children had the disease. One person trickled in, then another, until we had a total of twelve people. I remember the shock as the door kept opening to a new face every few minutes. I felt like an alien on earth, meeting my species for the first time. We ended up having people from all over the POTS spectrum—some wheelchair or walker bound and some with other related diseases like Ehlers-Danlos syndrome, mast cell activation disorders, intracranial hypertensions, and fibromyalgia.

I just wanted to cry. It was really the first time that I'd been in a room full of other people just like me, and you could see it in everyone's faces just how much they wanted and needed the support. I think we were all particularly grateful because we knew how hard it was to keep plans and make it to something like this when you're struggling with so many symptoms and challenges. I knew immediately that we were a like-minded group because the first attendee showed up wearing the exact same outfit as me! We joked that we were going to make everyone else feel awkward for not wearing the standard POTS uniform.

We looked over a PowerPoint of some different therapies and treatments and discussed who had tried what. We took our time, and talked for a few hours about how our lives had changed and what kind of impact the disease had on our families and relationships. This was an all-female group and most of the women brought their mothers or best friends, so they were also able to share their stories as caregivers.

There is a huge difference between the support you get online (which is also incredible) and the support you get in-person. Giving everyone a hug at the end of the night and interacting on a face-to-face level was so overwhelming. It was like being in a room full of best friends who knew you inside and out despite never having met you before. I was moved. This was one of the best moments I had experienced since I was diagnosed. Just the fact that there were other women at the meeting who were my age and were going through the exact same thing in their lives blew my mind.

Not all patients have good experiences with support groups, however. Travis Love, who shared his story about self-esteem and intimacy in an earlier chapter, also struggled to find the right balance of supporting others and being supported.

When I was first introduced to an MPS support system around my mid-teens, I was immediately turned off because it consisted mostly of bereaved parents or those with young children struggling to survive. I couldn't handle the constant neediness and depressing stories I heard every day. My condition wasn't as bad as theirs, and it was already tough enough to be the happy and optimistic guy that I was. I couldn't risk all the sadness and harsh realities of all those parents' stories dragging me down. I needed hope, so I avoided them.

For these groups to function at their best capacity, they need to have members that are willing to put in the work. "I can see that support groups can seem like a double-edged sword," says Travis. "You can either let them drag you down, or be the one pulling people up." It's important to remember that while support groups are there for you to find support, they can also be an unhealthy environment where misery goes to find more miserable company. The goal of a support group should always be to find ways, through the help of others, to move forward in life through your challenges. When you find people who have a similar goal of functioning beyond those challenges, you've found the right place. Certainly, the best way to ensure a good flow of helpful information is to make sure there is a designated leader in the group who is planning either activities or topics of conversation. You might seek out a group that meets at different locations, does different activities together, or pursues common interests.

Here are some tips for organizing your own, in-person support group. (For more extensive tips on starting a support group, you can download the online "Support Group Kit" at http://www.new harbinger.com/35999).

- Post the date and time of your meet-up in local forums and disease-specific forums.

- Get organized! Bring along any materials you want to share, such as information sheets, print-outs from the disease organization's website, and a sign-in sheet where attendees can list their name, number, and email to be alerted of the next meeting.

- Find a comfortable time and place to host the meeting. Try to organize the room in a way where all the chairs are facing toward a center, instead of one direction. You want to encourage a group conversation.

- Designate a leader to direct the conversations.

- Pre-pick topics to discuss.

- Make sure each attendee introduces themselves.

- Bring in local experts willing to share their expertise.

- Make sure an agreement of confidentiality between members is stated at each meeting.

- Send a follow-up email after the meeting to see if anyone had any thoughts or suggestions about the last meeting and if there was anything else they'd like to touch on during the next meeting.

- Don't be afraid to connect with attendees outside your meetings. Support groups are a great way to make friends with a lot in common!

Option 3: Mentors

Mentors don't have to be full-time support or even just one singular person who is committed to your situation alone. It can be a mentor from a support group or other patients who have gone down a similar road. You can find mentors in a variety of places, including in-person and online support groups, through friends and relatives, and even through your doctor if he's willing to forward your information on to another patient. The most important thing is that you feel comfortable going to them in times of turmoil to ask questions, seek advice, and find comfort.

Not long after I was first diagnosed with POTS, I got a phone call from an experienced patient. She explained that my mother had posted my story on a forum online and she'd asked for my number to get in touch. She said that she'd been diagnosed only a few years ago, but that she was sure she'd had this disease since childhood. "Do you still work?" I asked her. (I straddled the line of unemployment at that time, and that was one of my most burning questions.) She said, "Oh yeah, definitely. There's only been a few flares where I wasn't able to." I felt my heart do a backflip in my chest. I fired off more questions: "Do you take medications? Have you had any heart surgeries? Are you better off living in a colder climate?" She quickly answered all my questions, mostly optimistically. I continued with my line of questions. "Were you able to have kids?" I asked. "Three," she said, and I had to wipe the tears away. I said, "You didn't have any problems? You were fine?" She confessed, "I gave birth in the cardiac unit. I almost had a heart attack during labor, but they monitored me and I was okay."

She continued to explain that not everything was simple, but it was survivable. This conversation was so important to me because we can get mixed signals about what we may or may not be able to do in the future, especially from doctors who are trying to express how important it is that we take our diseases seriously. Hearing from another patient can help put your fears into perspective and open your eyes to options you didn't know you had. It was the first time since researching my diagnosis online that I started to feel optimistic.

Whether you're brainstorming medication options with another patient in the waiting room, or you're getting a call from a stranger who found your story online, these kinds of connections are a great way to start the process of getting educated about your disease. It can also help alleviate some of the fears you have about how your life will look. And, later, when you feel you've gotten a better grip on your disease, make sure to pay it forward to another newbie.

What Makes a Good Mentor?

- Someone who has balance in their own life, despite their condition

- The ability to break bad news gently

- Someone who has the time and knowledge to answer questions on living with the disease

Other Kinds of Support

Therapy

One support option you might consider is a more private one. One-on-one therapy can be a useful tool in the struggle to balance your daily life. Checking in with a licensed counselor once or more a week can give you an opportunity to vent, discuss setbacks and growth, and help you to make sense of your feelings.

Before I organized the first support group, I tried going to a therapist to develop some coping strategies. I'll admit, it took trying out several different psychologists before I found one I felt comfortable with. For me, psychoanalytical therapies that explored issues in my childhood were completely unhelpful for teaching me how to handle my problems. Sometimes venting about my stress felt like a relief, but when there was no constructive follow-up, it just made me feel more helpless. I needed action. I then discovered cognitive and behavioral therapies. This kind of therapy taught me to examine my roadblocks, set goals, and recognize progress. I also needed a very vocal therapist who would help pull me out of my shame or pity spirals and get me back on track. I did sessions on and off for about two years before I felt confident that I was on a good path to continue managing my disease on my own.

Therapy is available for free or at a reduced cost through multiple channels. I was fortunate enough to get a reduced rate from a local Jewish Community Center. You'll find that many other community and religious centers offer non-religious based counseling. You can also check with local universities who have programs for students training to be psychologists. Many insurance companies also cover therapy for a small co-pay. For patients who are homebound, there are also therapists who make themselves available online through Skype and other video-to-video programs.

Therapy is certainly a personal choice, and different kinds work for different patients. You may try exploring a few different types of therapy before settling on one treatment. Many psychologists are covered under major insurance plans, look for a therapist who is within your plan. Start by asking your insurance company for a list of psychologists in your zip code.

Professional and Academic Support

As we mentioned earlier, both schools and work places have rules to follow when it comes to providing safe and accommodating spaces for employees and students. Don't be afraid to reach out to your guidance counselor or HR representative for guidance on what accommodations are available to you.

Community Support

Neighbors, local government, and local non-profit organizations are all good support resources. (Well, maybe not all your neighbors, but hopefully you've got one or two that will help shovel the sidewalk when you're too weak to pick up a shovel.) Programs like Meals on Wheels can help you get nutritious food when you're unable to shop. Many county offices offer free or discounted transportation to patients.

Non-Profits

From patient education to assistance with medical bills, there are thousands of non-profit agencies across the country whose sole purpose is to help patients lead a more successful life. There are non-profits that help pay medical bills (such as, https://www.patientservicesinc.org), help you learn how to become a more empowered patient (such as, http://patientadvocate.org), and programs that can help to make medications more affordable (such as http://rxoutreach.org). Disease-specific non-profits can help with a variety of problems. For instance, those with Fabry disease can reach out to Fabry.org to help pay an odd utility bill since air-conditioning is a life-sustaining need for patients with temperature dysregulation. Do a little exploring online to see what non-profits might help to eliminate for certain disease-related challenges in your life.

Spiritual Support

Many churches, temples, and other places of worship provide clergy support for one-on-one counseling and support groups. Joining a bible study or prayer group can give you a new source of support that you may not have considered. These resources often provide these services at little to no charge. This is a possible option for patients without insurance to receive the counsel they need to cope with the challenges of their disease.

For faith-based individuals, turning to their religion during times of duress can provide great comfort and support. Embracing your spirituality can help you to cope with your situation, give meaning to your journey, and connect with others going through similar struggles during activities like group prayer.

It's Okay to Need Support

Whatever you choose as the channel to give and receive support, remember that the urge to connect with others in a similar situation as you is a natural thing. It doesn't mean you want to throw yourself a pity party and it doesn't mean you need to share your most intimate thoughts. At the heart of a support system is an avenue to give yourself the opportunity to grow and learn from others.

Check in with your designated disease organization for a list of local support groups and professionals. For patients without a diagnosis, you can still turn to organizations like SWAN (Syndromes Without a Name) to find local support. Once you've established an effective outlet for coping with the stress of your disease, you'll be better equipped to deal with the real challenge of being a prepared patient.

CHAPTER 7

The World Won't Wait: School and Work

If you've grown up with your disease, it won't be a huge surprise that your education, career, and social life will be another thing that's massively affected. At some point, you'll start to witness a pattern develop in your life. You'll feel well, so you have more energy. That energy helps you do well at work because you're able to focus on your projects and not your symptoms. Success at the workplace then leads to a balanced social life, which then leads you to start making plans for the future. Then this happens: Something (a meal, stress, a missed medication, a new medication) triggers your symptoms, your energy decreases, you start to do poorly at work because you have to reserve your energy to do everyday tasks, you have no available energy for friends or your partner, and you get depressed and stop making plans for your future. As you become consumed by the feeling of having the rug pulled out from under you, you realize that despite your entire world falling apart, life is still going on around you, without you!

After a relapse like this, it's a mad scramble to pick yourself up again, catch up on your schoolwork and your responsibilities, and check in with all the people you have relationships with. In the midst of picking up the pieces after relapse, you also have to carry the incredibly inconvenient burden of knowing that you can *push, run,* and *hang on* for dear life, but the reality is that you will never be capable of living a life uninterrupted by illness. Heavy, right?

For me, this epiphany came in two waves. The first emotion was an incredible sadness. The life I had hoped to live was forever changed. I could no longer ignore that some of my life goals would now have to be altered. The second emotion, however, was incredible relief. Fully understanding the limitations of my disease and starting to envision a more realistic and functional life plan gave me a reprieve from the dark cloud of uncertainty. There's just no room for improvement in life without accepting the idea that we must respond to each new crisis in a comfortable and effective way, instead of fighting against it until we've exhausted ourselves.

It's a natural reaction to want to grieve the life you wanted had you been born into that "perfect" body. You may feel sadness when the door is shutting on some of the paths you wanted to take. It's also a natural reaction to realize that you can be honest about your future without completely losing your hope, happiness, and sanity. It's okay to feel relieved that you no longer need to rise to the expectations that repel the reality of your condition. Once you get to this moment in your journey, you can start to realistically plan and prepare to live a meaningful life.

When it comes to exploring options for your future, it's important to keep an open mind. Your timelines may be different from others, and your roads a little less traveled. We've talked about how to halt our guilt, go about making new friends (and keeping old ones), build social networks, and create your elevator pitch. It can also help to know that by admitting and accepting your limitations, you can now create the life you want.

Going to School

As a high school student, if I wasn't high-tailing it to class in between bathroom breaks or explaining my absences to everyone from guidance counselors to teachers, I was somewhere in the nurse's office, trying to untangle the very complicated storyline of my undiagnosed disease. I was a hot mess.

Traditional schooling isn't designed for those who haven't learned to manage their disease. Who the hell ever learned to manage their disease while still in high school? Trying to "get by" without assistance from your school's faculty and staff is nearly impossible. It's important to set appointments with your school's disability program coordinator and discuss your options for schooling. Start by calling your school's guidance counselor. Students are generally divided between different counselors by last name, so check with the front office staff to guide you to the right one. When you're able to get a meeting with them, make sure you come prepared. Bring the following with you:

- Documentation from your doctor showing proof of your disease and what activities the disease might affect (sports, attendance, etc.).

- An idea of what sort of accommodations you'd like to request. You might want to request an elevator pass so you don't have to climb stairs. Or, you might want to ask that your teachers seat you in the front of the classroom so that you can see the board better. You can also ask for extensions on projects, leniency with attendance, and information on how to deal with an escalation of symptoms and how it would affect school work.

- A list of questions to ask about what the school's policies are that might affect you. Do they allow students to bring lunch from home to avoid possible food allergy triggers? Can a student with visual disabilities bring a laptop or other device to help with eye strain during lessons? Can a student leave a classroom without permission if they have an emergency?

- An emergency contact list with your parents' information and any others who have signed permission agreements that allow them to pick you up from school in case you get ill in the middle of the day.

- Any past documentation from your current or previous schools.

During my freshman year of high school, I ended up being part of a program called Hospital Homebound (HH). This was in an era where we were still getting used to using the internet for everything. My classes were held through conference calls with my teachers and a few other students, and my assignments were emailed or mailed in. Since then, getting an education outside of the classroom is a whole new world. Virtual school is now available for middle schoolers, high schoolers, college students, and those who want to take continuing education courses. They can be done in your spare time, and on your own schedule in the comfort of your bedroom, living room, or hospital room. Your local school district should be able to offer you information on how to register for their online programs.

Since I had dropped out of one or two classes during my sophomore year, unable to find a balance between absences and coursework, I was able to re-take classes through a virtual school on the weekends or at night. By my senior year of high school, the year I was most debilitated by my disease, I felt like I had exhausted all my options. I was in advanced classes that I needed to sit through the lectures for. I was falling behind on all my assignments. I was only able to stay conscious for about four hours each day. It usually took me an hour to wake up, get ready, eat breakfast, and get to my first class, which then only left me with three hours. Since my first period class was two hours, that gave me only half of one other class I could sit through.

When I went to see my principal about this, I said, "I need help. I need to graduate on time and I need to get through all my classes. I can't stay awake and this isn't working." Mr. Licata wanted to help me the best that he could and asked me what would work best for me. I told him, "My AP English final paper is a beast. I need to be in the workshop with my teacher in the morning. I'm going to have a math tutor in the mornings on the weekend so I can get those classes taken care of, and the rest of my classes need to send me home with the reading material and the assignments. I can only be on campus for three hours a day. Max."

The school had a lot of restrictions on absences and attendance. Technically they were supposed to fail students who missed seventy-five percent or more of their scheduled classes. But after I pleaded my case, they made an exception. A meeting was called with my teachers. They were asked to make themselves available to me by email, to allow me to hand in my assignments in the mornings, and to have new material waiting for me to pick up. I finished my final paper in English and for the rest of the year managed to make it to bed unscathed every day before noon.

None of this would have been possible if I didn't ask. Learning how and when to ask for help is going to be a huge asset to you in life. When it comes to sustaining a sense of normalcy and promoting the likelihood of your success, asking for help is the most responsible thing you can do.

Making an Education Plan

Let's talk about the system that's already in place for students in need. A 504/IEP plan is an individualized educational plan designed to support students with disabilities. Even if you're not missing a limb or legally blind, this plan can still cover you. It's individualized for your needs.

Your 504 Plan/IEP is your responsibility. You're going to be standing on the front porch for a long time if you never knock. To receive the benefits and allowances of a disability plan, you need to ask for it! For students with invisible disabilities like Crohn's disease, fibromyalgia, chronic fatigue, lupus, and narcolepsy, your school will be less inclined to go out of its way to make sure you're on the plan. You will need to go to your guidance counselor as early in the school year as possible and ask to set up a plan.

What Will Your School Define as a Disability?

In 2009, the Americans with Disabilities Act of 2008 came into effect. It stated that the definition of disability had to include those who demonstrated symptoms that substantially limited a "major life activity." According to this act, symptoms can also fluctuate between active and inactive and still be termed a disability, even when the symptom does not impact the learning process. These included:

- Sleeping: For students whose fatigue cuts days short.

- Standing: For students who may not have the stamina for oral reports, field trips, or lines.

- Eating: For students with time-sensitive feeding schedules, feeding tubes, or other GI issues.

- Lifting: For students who cannot carry their books or lug around backpacks.

- Reading: For students who need to sit closer to the front of the class, or need translation, braille, or other forms of visual support.

- Concentrating: For students who need extra time to process materials.

- Breathing: For students who need breaks for nebulizer or inhaler use, or need to stay away from areas of the school with allergens or mold.

- Hearing: For students who need help with audio support.

- Seeing: For students who need help with visual support.

- Communicating: For students who need translators or other forms of communication support.

- Walking: For students who need to use accessible parts of the campus.

The fact is that it behooves your school to see you graduate. Having another drop-out reflects poorly on them. Be open and realistic with your academic advisors about the severity and complexity of your disease. Walk them through a day in your life and see what small and manageable adjustments can be made to make things a little easier for you. Eventually, if your illness progresses to a point where attending school is no longer possible, your counselors and advisors should be able to guide and assist you by getting you into an alternative schooling option.

Tips for a Conscious Education Plan in High School and College

1. **Start seeing your advisors early and often.** Allow them to walk you through your entire schedule of intended

courses over the next few years. You don't want to make the mistake of wasting time with unnecessary classes.

2. **Try to schedule more intense classes during periods with less intense symptoms.** (If your allergies are more irritated in the winter, plan your more advanced courses in the spring.)

3. **Don't be afraid to try different educational alternatives.** Summer school, virtual school, and home schooling are all great options for those who may not be able to fit a full school day into their schedules or energy budget.

4. **Remember that nothing is ever set in stone.** You may feel that some schools have an inflexible attitude towards attendance or deadlines, but you'd be surprised how much they can help you work with the tides of your disease.

5. **Start from the top down.** When a crisis hits and you need an immediate and drastic change in your educational plan, don't start with your teachers, start with your school's administration. Make an appointment with the principal; they may be able to help bend certain rules to get you through the semester.

6. **Be a part of the team.** Your attitude towards your education is what matters most. All the exceptions in the world can be made for you, but if you don't have the desire or drive to get through school, you will not succeed. Promise your educational team that you're in this for the long haul, that you're as committed to the success of your education as they are, and that you're going to take full advantage of the leeway they've given you to focus on your school work.

Managing a Career and Employment

When you transition from student to employee, you will probably encounter less support. The first step is to think long and hard about what kind of employment best suits your abilities. By the age of sixteen, few people realize that they'll probably never be able to work a nine-to-five job. The normal course of employment just isn't an option for patients with life-limiting illnesses. Setting realistic goals for their careers is something that needs to be taken on with out-of-the-box thinking. The good news is that technology has moved us into an age where your desk doesn't necessarily have to be in the same building as your co-workers to do your job. Building the necessary skill set to be a work-from-home employee, consultant, or self-employed professional is possible. There are also many adjustments for disabilities that can be negotiated in standard workplaces. In this section, we'll cover some of the ways you can secure the best accommodations for your needs at your workplace.

Expectations about Your Career

Is a person with rheumatoid arthritis going to be a massage therapist? Is a patient with ulcerative colitis going to have a stupendous career as a food reviewer? What about someone with chronic fatigue—do you think they'd be a quick hire as a physical education teacher? I'm not writing this to slay your spirit or crush your dream, but you're in for a rude awakening if you expect to go forth into the night with your spandex and your cape jumping from one fire escape to another with inflamed tendons. It's important for your physical and emotional well-being to test your limits regarding what kind of job you can handle. Want to be a cop? Do a ride-along for a few days to see if you can handle the pace. Want to be a teacher? Assist in the classroom for a few weeks to see if the responsibility of managing students is too much for you. Want to be a food reviewer? Ask for the chef's specialty without asking if it has wheat, dairy, or shellfish in it.

For patients who discover their diagnosis earlier on in life, there's a great chance they'll be able to avoid massive disappointment and turmoil by translating their career goals into something achievable. But what if your disease hits you in the middle of med school or just as you got that promotion you've been shooting for all year? Some think of it the way a cancer patient chooses to shave their head before chemo. They know now that something is happening and that to live and have a less painful life, they need to have this therapy. This therapy will cause them to lose all their hair. It's either going to happen the easy (and potentially less terrifying) way, or they're going to watch clumps of their hair fall out in the shower every night until they're bald.

In your situation, you can choose to fight against the tides of your disease and drag yourself through your work day with all the stress and anxiety it will cause, or you can choose to accept a change in pace and profession and move on. It may not seem like you're making a career choice when it comes to chronic illness and employment, but you are. Neither of these choices are wrong and not everyone with a chronic illness chooses to give up their day job, even if it means spending ten hours a day on their feet. Some patients' illnesses can be managed to the point where they can live a completely normal life. But most patients' lives revolve around flare-ups and remission.

You may begin to ask yourself: When will a flare-up strike next? What will I do if I can't call in sick? What happens to my insurance if I'm fired? Will my job really take me back when I'm well again? Having a disease doesn't mean lowering your expectations about your career, but instead expecting a different skill set from yourself. People with chronic illness contribute to the well-being of the world every day. They help people, employ people, and even run businesses from their hospital beds. There are so many jobs that can be done from the relative comfort of your own bedroom.

The following are some examples of jobs you can do online:

Marketing, Promotions, and Advertising. Are you a creative type? There are many opportunities to be part of a company's wing of marketing from your home base. Many employees teleconference in to team meetings, and send material back and forth over email.

Creative Writing and Copy Writing. If you've got a knack for the written word, you may be able to land a gig as a copywriter. Copywriters come in all shapes and sizes. You could find yourself writing content for anything from the back of shampoo bottles to paid posts on different lifestyle websites.

Video Editing and Graphic Design. Do you have skills in this technical field? With the right software on your computer to do editing and design, most of these positions are done as a freelancer or from home.

Appointment Setting and Virtual Personal Assistant. There is a whole world out there of employees and contractors who work from home. Consider teaming up with one of these experienced workers and acting as their virtual secretary.

Social Media Management and Community Liaison. With the rise of social media like Facebook, Twitter, Instagram, Pinterest, and LinkedIn, many companies hire one person devoted to interacting with their audience, answering questions, and forwarding complaints or concerns to the right department.

Tutoring and Teaching Online Classes or Instructional Videos. Did you know you can make a living teaching others about some of your favorite subjects through video sharing sites like YouTube and Vimeo? These people teach everything from how to apply a sexy eyeliner to how to build Ikea furniture.

Science, Medicine, and Technology. Contrary to popular belief, there are positions for professionals in these fields that involve telecommuting. In recent years, there have been great advancements that allow doctors to see patients through video conferencing. Many pharmaceutical companies employ legions of nurses to answer phone calls related to patient concerns. Doctors, nurses, and scientists are also in great demand as consultants for new diagnostic technology, medical apps, tutoring, and teaching.

These are just a few ideas! Keep in mind that there is always a way to have a meaningful, fulfilling career with an active chronic illness; it just takes time, determination, and planning.

Four Basic Rules for Dealing with Your Disease and Your Career

Rule #1: Nobody Needs to Know Your Business Unless You Tell Them

There's a long list of people you don't have to talk about your disease with. Your employer or potential employer is on that list. Legally you don't have to disclose anything about your disease. The Americans with Disabilities Act prohibits discrimination against people with disabilities in employment, transportation, public accommodation, communications, and governmental activities. You don't need to mention it on your resume or even in your interview. And, hey, if your illness never has and never will affect your job performance, you go on with your bad self, baby! Nobody needs to know your business. But before you try to shove that bag of saline and IV pain killers in your purse, ask yourself one question: Am I being a moron?

If your disease is plainly, obviously, and inevitably going to get in the way of your work responsibilities, you need to seriously assess where, how, and to whom you're going to be disclosing that information.

Ask yourself the following questions:

- Do my symptoms ever interfere with my work projects?

- Do I sometimes need days, weeks, or even entire months off because of out-of-control flare-ups?

- Does my high-pain level mean I might be at a higher risk to lose my temper with a rude customer?

- Do my sleep attacks make me an unfortunate candidate to drive the school bus?

- As a flight attendant, during a possible plane crash, will all the passengers die on the plane because they didn't get directions on how to attach their oxygen masks because I was in the bathroom with the runs associated with my chronic disease?

- Does my immune deficiency disease mean that my position as a secretary at a pediatrician's office is probably a very bad, germ-ridden idea?

If you think your disease might impact your job performance down the road, you should think about saying something. You might say something like, "I have narcolepsy, which means I'm going to have to create my schedule around my fatigue until I can find a treatment that works well for me. I'm happy to take some work home for nights and weekends to make up for time missed." This is also a good time to whip out your elevator speech. However, even though it violates the protection you should receive under the ADA, you can't do a single thing if a company eliminates you in their search for an employee because of your illness. They can just blame it on something else, like not enough experience.

Rule #2: You Don't Have the Luxury, So Deal with It

Unlike many other people your age and in your field, you do not have the luxury of slacking off, being a bad employee, or not working hard at your job. This is just another fact of life under the umbrella of accepting your chronic illness. The truth is that you will always have to work hard because you need a job that has health insurance and enough financial stability to support your medical bills and other expenses related to the disease. The good news is that when you're good at what you do, and it's something you like to do, the hard work is worth it.

Rule #3: Do Something You're Good at and Something You Like

Do something you love and that you're good at. This will make the long days, the bad days, the days where you need to push yourself to make it through the hard stuff, more tolerable. You may be thinking that's not realistic: "Will I have to work a shit job because no one would possibly hire someone like me to do a job I love?" As in all areas of life, this is another area to practice self-love. What's the worst thing that could happen if you go for the gold?

You did not lose the privilege to be loved when you got sick. You did not lose the privilege to be treated with respect. You did not lose the privilege to work toward a job that gives you meaning. It does not always mean you will work the exact job that you want, but you can certainly gear your search toward the kind of career you'd ultimately aspire to. Take your time. Think about where your skills are most needed. What do you have to offer? Your body may not be what it once was, but there's more to you than just a broken body.

Rule #4: Accommodate Yourself

This rule is about realizing that the only person who can make you comfortable in your life is *you*. Ask for the quiet office that will give you space and serenity to work through the intolerable early start of migraines. The only person who knows what you really need is you. So, ask for those flexible hours. You control whether you sit or stand. Take a break every two hours, or for two minutes every hour.

Take care of yourself by either taking it easy or asking for things to make your life easier. You can ask for things like an upgraded desk chair for back pain, to work your last few hours of the day from home, or to stay a little later at work so you can take off a little earlier the next day. There are a lot of changes that can be made to accommodate your needs. When you choose a job that you are qualified for and are good at, it's okay to ask for help. Companies want to keep good employees, and good employees can usually be found at companies that honor their requests for a comfortable work environment.

Rule #5: Plan for the Worst-Case Scenario

Some people are alarmists. Some people are hoarders. Some people have nuclear fallout shelters underneath their kid's tree house. I'm not saying you should be any of these people. I'm just saying that you should have a healthy sense of reality when it comes to your job security.

Here's a truth for you: Remission is a blissful period where your life comes together in all the empty places. Here's another truth for you: Chronic doesn't mean "just that one time." Prepare for that worst-case scenario. Prepare for the idea that you could lose your job because your illness might return. It can happen. Some ways to prepare are: continuously updating your resume with new skills, always being on the lookout for jobs that allow you to telecommute or create your own hours, or talking to your boss about accommodations *before* your flare-up.

Frequently Asked Questions: Working with an Invisible Chronic Illness

You probably have been in many scenarios already where you've felt confused about when, where, and with whom you need to share your disease details with. What are your rights? In general, what is the right thing to do? Below are some frequently asked questions regarding the workplace and your disease.

When should I tell my potential employer about my chronic illness?

This is a frequently asked question and the answer is, well, that depends. Will your illness affect your job performance? Depending on the sort of job you have, you may not have to tell your employer at all. If you feel that even through a difficult flare-up of symptoms you could still complete your work to the best of your ability, then it's no one's business but your own. However, if you feel that there is a chance you could seriously impact the quality of your company or even your co-worker's jobs, then you do have a responsibility to be upfront about your illness. Even if you do feel compelled to explain your illness, make sure to come forward with a plan of contingency on how you will make sure your job performance isn't affected, such as training another employee to take over in case of an emergency, or being willing to perform job tasks over the phone or online from home.

My illness is out of control right now, but I have the opportunity to take on a job. Should I go for it or turn it down?

When opportunity knocks, it can be totally soul-crushing to shut the door in its face. At the same time, you need to be realistic about what you can handle. If you're constantly in and out of the hospital and this opportunity requires a strict schedule that you have to abide by, you may have to turn it down. The trick to keeping those doors open is to make strong connections with those who are offering you the opportunity. Be honest with them about your condition and say that even though you feel they're right, and you would be the perfect person for the position, you're just not physically capable of doing this job without accommodations. You'd be surprised, but many times a pragmatic explanation will not only help to kick open the door, it will roll out the red carpet with benefits and allowances.

As a freelancer, there have been multiple month-long periods where I've just had to say, "no thanks" even when I was *hurting* for the money. Most of the time the jobs were still waiting for me when I got better, and other times I was referred from those who had needed me in the past to friends or associates that needed my help now. Better to save your reputation as a good (but hard to come by) consultant, than as a flaky one.

Can I be fired for having a chronic illness?

Employees in the United States are generally offered nine paid sick days a year. Obviously, if you have a chronic illness and a full time, in-office job, that's probably not going to being enough sick days by a long shot. Do you have protection against discrimination and surprises? Sure. The Americans with Disabilities Act forces employers to make adjustments for disabled workers, usually with time off. The Family and Medical Leave Act gives you up to twelve weeks off without pay each year for medical emergencies.

But your chronic illness probably isn't an emergency. I get it. Life is tough with a chronic illness, but it's your life now. So, cry a little, suck it up, and start planning a more successful life with your disease. If you know you have a chronic illness, then be preventative by not surprising your employer by suddenly taking twelve weeks off with no notice of your disease. Don't leave your company hanging by a thread because you never took the time to prepare your co-workers or employer for your absence. Your disease is your responsibility now and you can choose to build an infrastructure to support it or you can deal with the consequences when things begin to fall apart.

How to Organize Your Life When Your Illness is a Full-Time Job

These days, my plate is very full. I've even had to turn down clients for work. I keep asking myself, why is it that I'm always short on time and energy? What do I do all day that is keeping me so busy and distracted? I sometimes forget that my disease is a full-time job. I have cardiac rehab three times a week, the infusion center on Tuesday, and the standing doctor's appointment on Thursday. If there are any little gaps in my calendar, you'll find me face down on my desk trying to figure out how to squeeze in a nap between press releases. The consequences of missing work because of a flare-up are real. If I don't work, I won't get paid, which means I can't pay for rent, car insurance, or groceries. If I don't take care of my disease by going to cardiac rehab, getting my IVs on schedule, or taking my medicine, I'll get sick, be hospitalized, and lose all the freedoms and privileges of my normal life.

In high school and college, you might be able to get your classes and teachers to work with you, but the real world has no 504 plan and you've got to learn to maximize your energy to earn money, sustain relationships, and organize your life. I find myself in enough hospital rooms and unintentional napping scenarios that I wouldn't rush to call myself an expert on a perfect life with chronic illness, but I've got a few tricks up my sleeve I can share. Having my own schedule, guidelines, and privileges means that I can work around my illness—from the hospital bed and home. There are millions of other people who also work like this. Here are some tips on how to balance a chronic illness with a busy life and work schedule.

Work from Home

Telecommuting is the way to go. This is what they invented Skype for. Let your employer know that you're struggling to concentrate at the office and that you feel the quality of your work would improve if you were able to work from home during periods of illness. Let them know you have reliable internet and phone access and will be able to carry on your current projects with constant communication with the rest of the staff via phone and email.

Prevent Flare-ups

Prevention of flare-ups is less time-consuming than having them constantly. With chronic illness, the more run down you become, the harder it is to manage your daily life. It's important to do everything possible to stop a symptom before it starts. For example, you might consider ways to prevent joint pain by investing in a cart to help you carry heavy groceries and ease the physical burden. If you have a gastrointestinal disorder, you may want to keep "safe" foods in the pantry, just so you can always have the option of making a reasonable meal choice.

Don't Take It Too Seriously

If you miss an event or you're too tired to do something, don't beat yourself up over it. There's always another day. There's always tomorrow. You fail a class? That's life. You'll do better next semester.

Have a Few Irons in the Fire

At some point, we all fall. When we do, it's a good idea to not need to rely on a single project, job, or paycheck. Working from home gives you the opportunity to manage multiple opportunities. Find a way to manage them.

Keep an Agenda

If I don't write down an appointment in my calendar, I will forget about it. I've completely missed out on important events when I forgot to write them down in my calendar. Chronic illness has a way of compromising plans. I tend to try and fit in a nap or relaxation/down time whenever there's a gap in my calendar. The worst is waking up from a nap to realize you forgot a conference call.

Save for a Monsoon

Forget a rainy day! With a chronic illness, you never know when you're going to be down for the count. Start putting away part of every paycheck into savings. Live beneath your means. Try to always have an emergency fund for those crappy weeks when you just can't do it.

Securing Accommodations at Work

If you already have a job that you don't want to leave, you can talk to your employer about making adjustments for your illness so you can continue working. Some possible accommodations might include:

- Being able to take more breaks

- Working part-time from home

- Being allowed to choose your own hours, or cut back on your hours

- Moving to a better office for your condition (more/less cold air, fewer stairs, one with a couch where you can rest, etc.)

- Being able to make up hours when you have a doctor's appointment during work hours

- Being able to Skype-in to important meetings instead of traveling to meet clients

Don't be afraid to think outside the box. You need to do what you have to do. If that means buying an air mattress and setting it up in your office so you can sleep during your lunch hour, then that's what you need to do. If that means paying a co-worker to drive you home at the end of the day, in case you're too tired to concentrate, then that's what you need to do. Maybe you need to put a drape in your cubicle to block out the sun if it's causing you migraines, or buy a foot massager for underneath your desk if you need an escape from the pain. You have a living to make. Don't be ashamed of doing what you need to do to survive.

Alternative Employment Strategies

When working full-time is not an option, there are still more solutions. The trick is to play to your strengths and try to find a job that compliments your skill set. Joan Friedlander, author of *Business from Bed: The 6-Step Comeback Plan to Get Yourself Working After a Health Crisis* (2012) lived for years with a rather crippling case of Crohn's disease, yet now works from home as a freelance author and coach. Crohn's disease put a big dent in my sense of confidence and well-being," says Friedlander.

> *It took several years of trial and error, but I was eventually able to recover that same sense of purpose and direction I felt as a training manager, through coaching, teaching, and writing. Furthermore, I had to figure out how to earn a good living, doing work I love in a way that supports my well-being. It has meant breaking with the traditional rules of business to find my own pathway to success. No matter your age or your life's circumstances, the question about how to earn a good living doing work you enjoy is an important one. After all, we live in a world where health and well-being depend on it. Some people work for money, some for the joy of the work itself, and others because they're called to a mission that won't let go. As you contemplate success on this material plane, why not include capacity and ease? Because whatever job you are doing, you should be able to do it—or at least the important tasks—even on your worst day (from your toilet, hospital bed, on heavy medication, etc.).*

For some, ease looks like a nine-to-five job; for others, it's a telecommuting gig or perhaps even owning their own business. Friedlander asks: "What if you could spend most of your working time doing work that is as 'natural' as breathing? What might that look like, feel like?" For me, what wore me out the most was having to visit clients in person. I could talk for hours on the telephone. I could write long, detailed, and clear emails. But, sitting through a meeting in formal business clothes trying to hide every tremor and migraine was exhausting. I just couldn't keep up the act. I remember walking out of an investor meeting for one of my PR clients one afternoon and just sitting in my car trying to peel off my jacket that I'd soaked in sweat from stress. In my visor mirror I looked pale and my make-up was gone. But the thing that I saw most clearly in that moment was that I was so unhappy. This wasn't how I wanted to spend my days. Why was I torturing myself doing something that didn't support everything my body was telling me it needed? Wasn't there another way?

There is. Finding out that telecommuting was an option was half the battle. The other half was allowing myself the freedom to take advantage of it. I think I felt like working entirely from home was a way of giving up. It took time for me to realize that adjusting my career to better fit my health wasn't giving up, but rather putting my health first. I knew that if I could do that, I was ultimately making a better decision for my career in the long term. Taking the focus off my physical limitations meant that I could work on more complex projects for longer hours and with less stress. Letting my clients and employers know what was going on with my health led to more understanding and accommodations, and fewer excuses on my part. Taking a real, hard look at how my disease was affecting my career was a bitter pill to swallow, but without doing so I would never have been able to change things for the better.

Disability

You've probably thought about it. Is it possible that your illness qualifies as a full-time job at this point? Do you need government assistance to pay your bills and live your life? How does the process of securing disability work? Do you need a lawyer? These are all very common questions for patients staring down the application for Social Security Disability Benefits.

What is Disability?

Disability Social Security is a collection of services and benefits made specifically for those who cannot work because of a life-limiting illness. About eight million Americans are currently on disability. The benefits include:

Supplemental Security Income: This is the amount of funds issued to a patient each month to help them with living expenses they could not otherwise afford due to their inability to work full-time with their disease.

Social Security Disability Insurance: In most situations, if a person is eligible for Social Security, they are also eligible for a program called Medicaid. Medicaid is insurance that helps pay medical expenses.

Social Services: Those who are approved for disability may qualify to receive homecare, transportation, and food delivery services.

Interim Assistance Payments: This is when a person receives funds from Social Security while they wait to be approved for Social Security. The money given from these payments will be deducted from future benefits if the person is approved.

Social Nutrition Assistance Program (SNAP): Formerly known as food stamps, SNAP helps to pay for groceries.

Applying for Disability

Though the initial process of applying for disability is simply filling out a form, many patients find the rest of the process to be difficult. First you must assess whether you qualify for the service. The Social Security Administration lists the following as requirements to qualify:

To receive disability, you must have been disabled for at least five months.

Your condition must result in the inability to do any substantial gainful activity that can be expected to result in death, or has lasted or can be expected to last for a continuous period of no less than twelve months.

If you have more specific questions about your particular situation, there are Social Security offices in your area. You can call, make an appointment, and have someone walk you through the process and paperwork. They can also help to tell you if there are more programs in your community that might be able to help you. You can learn how to apply in your state through https://ssa.gov.

Staying One Step Ahead

At the end of the day, it's about creativity. It's about outsmarting your symptoms and being ready and waiting with a plan when they come barreling around the corner. You're already at an advantage, because you know what's coming. It feels like independence is always out of reach until we take the leap. Even then, there will be setbacks. Though there will be challenges, it is possible to remain independent. We've discussed how to choose jobs that fit your strengths, passions, and limitations and ways to make school a more progressive experience. In the next chapter, we'll look at some strategies for remaining independent once you've secured a sustainable school, work, and social life.

CHAPTER 8

Remaining Independent

Do you feel like "Can you do me a favor?" has become your catch-phrase? Do you feel like you're always in need of help to do even the simplest things? It can be frustrating, humiliating, and demeaning. You wonder how continuously asking for support will affect your relationships with other people. Will they come to resent you or expect you to always be incapable of providing for yourself? Relying on others for everything gets old and eventually you wear out your welcome. Will you ever regain independence?

Not long after I moved out of my parents' house I developed a pesky little condition called postural orthostatic tachycardia syndrome, which meant that as soon as I stood up from a sitting position, my pulse would quicken dramatically and my blood pressure would plummet. Sometimes my vision would black out completely before slowly returning. This resulted in many an episode of lying face down on my floor, waiting for my blood to begin circulating again and my vision to come back.

If I had known I would have spells like this during the endless months of apartment hunting, I probably would have never moved out of my parents' house. Just the thought of being completely alone and helpless, unable to get myself to the hospital, or with nobody around to get me help, was terrifying. But, once I was on my own, I learned that without help I could still survive. I stood up. I dropped down. I laid on my floor for about five minutes trying to figure out what my next move was. I reached up and felt around for my cell phone on my nightstand. I crawled over to my dog's bed and laid down on it. I called my mom and then waited there for her to pick me up. And, I lived.

You will survive something like this too. Whether it's your mother, friend, or EMT who picks you up off the floor, or you manage to get up again with the help of assistive devices you've had installed, your dog is not going to eat your face. You will be way too prepared for an emergency landing to let that happen.

While there are certainly extreme situations in which you can't be alone and help yourself, it doesn't mean you can't create safeguards to help you remain independent. Planning is key to a more predictable life with chronic illness. Your doctors won't be able to tell you when the next flare will strike, but if you start preparing for it now, there's little to worry about when it arrives. Knowing you've planned for the potential outcomes of your symptoms is a responsible move, an almost freeing one. Even if things don't pan out perfectly, you've made an active attempt to prepare. You've taken control over what small things you do have control over.

You'll find that your little safeguards have a huge impact on your work, social life, education, and relationships. Instead of landing you in sticky situations with angry bosses and disappointed friends, you'll encounter understanding and respect for your ability to show up despite your adversities. While it's great to please those around you and maintain those jobs and relationships, what's the point if they don't ultimately lead to your independence as a person? Plan for your job to be interrupted. Plan for your dates to be canceled. Just don't forget to plan for *you*—your happiness and your right to live where and with whom you want to live. This chapter will help you evaluate if you are ready to go out on your own and provide some examples of how to establish the groundwork for autonomy in your adult life.

Are You Ready for Independence?

Here are some things to contemplate before taking the big leap of independence. Start by asking yourself the following questions:

Can I handle the day-to-day management of my disease? Are you going to the hospital a little too frequently? Have you been able to get yourself to and from doctors' appointments, get your medications, and address issues in a safe amount of time?

Can I afford this? Beyond the usual responsibilities of independent living, like rent, utilities, car insurance, car payments, gas, or public transport costs, you'll have the burden of additional financial problems. These include insurance premiums, appointment and prescription co-pays, fees for alternative therapies, and the upgraded cost of specialty foods like gluten-free products.

Am I physically capable of independent living? If not, can I afford or get the help I need to make it all possible? Take a moment to really think on this one. Will you be able to clean your home, go out and stock your fridge with groceries, take care of your pets, prepare your own meals, and manage your bills alone? If not, can you afford to pay someone to help you do these things? Or trade something with a friend or neighbor to get their help for free? Review chapter 6 again and think about your support structure. Can any of these resources provide help?

What is my back-up plan if things don't work? Can you break your lease without an unaffordable financial penalty? Can you move back in with your parents? Will you be able to obtain government funding for living expenses if you can no longer work? It's depressing to consider these possibilities, but it's better to think about the solutions for these situations now, rather than during a crisis.

The first step toward independence is taking a risk. Even though it could end badly, if you set yourself up for success, it's worth it. The next step is coming face-to-face with your biggest fears around autonomy.

Address Your Biggest Fears with Easy Solutions

In the days before I moved out of my parents' house, I found myself pacing the hallway between our bedrooms. I was remembering all the times I'd shout out for my mother to come help me in the middle of the night when I couldn't move or something had gone terribly wrong. It would only take her a minute to get to me and I would know that I was safe. I was feeling so much fear about leaving her. I wanted and needed to move out and start my life, but I also had to address my fears first.

Fear #1: Help! I've Fallen and I Can't Get Up!

There are plenty of preventative measures you can take to make sure you don't end up laying on your floor for three days, including:

- **Living with a Roommate:** Whether it's a friend or a significant other, not living completely alone can be an unimaginably huge source of comfort. Even if they're not your main caretaker, just having another body in the house means they'll be able to help you out of tricky situations.

- **Using a Life Alert® System:** Hey, it worked for the lady in the commercial! But seriously, Life Alert® and systems like it can be valuable to those who are sick and unsteady on their feet. There are systems that can connect you to an operator who can give you the choice of calling an ambulance or a family member.

- **Keeping Your Cell on You at All Times:** While I don't always have mine in my back pocket, I do make sure to always bring my phone with me whenever I go, just in case of emergency. I don't want to have to climb up the stairs if I'm having a physical emergency.

Fear #2: Can I Stay Healthy Enough to Keep My Job?

This was the number one question I received through my blog last year, and it is understandably a common fear. Here are some suggestions on how you can plan to help keep your job:

- **Begin Saving:** While it won't always be realistic to save ninety percent of your paycheck, start putting away as much as you can bear to live without. Even if you're just throwing twenty dollars here and there into your online savings account, it starts to add up.

- **Have a Financial Support System and Be Responsible About It:** When it came to taking money from friends and family, I felt ashamed. But, the idea of living at home with my parents until I was forty was just as shameful. When push came to shove, if I needed to borrow money, I did. As soon as I could, I paid back what I owed.

- **Have a Credit Card and Good Credit:** It's not like you can snap your fingers and instantly have all those medical debts removed from your credit report. You can't go back in time and erase the month you were late on rent because you were in the hospital and unable to get out of bed. But working on creating good credit or mending bad credit should be a priority for you. At the end of the day, you may just not have the funds to support the extra financial burden that comes with having a chronic disease.

- **Check Your Company's Rules and Your Employee Rights:** Not sure if your sick days will cover the amount of days in which you may be sick? Speak with your company's HR person and try to create some preventative measures to help you stay employed. You may be able to work from home on certain days, or you may be able to take an extended leave. What you won't want to do is start considering these resources *after* you've already used up your sick days and your employer's patience and good will.

Fear #3: What If I Have Nothing In the House to Eat and I'm Too Fatigued to Make It to the Grocery Store and Back?

You stock up: frozen meals, canned meals, etc. I even keep a couple of individual bags of Chex™ Mix in my upstairs bathroom cabinets just in case I can't make it downstairs and I need to eat something filling with my medication. If I've run out of my stockpile, I can always get a delivery from a local restaurant or call in a favor from a friend who can pick me up something. You can't always rely on greasy take-out though, so you may consider making and freezing some healthier meals to keep on hand.

Fear #4: I'm Scared I Won't Be Able to Handle the Stress on My Own

Are you really on your own? If you can still reach out to family, friends, co-workers, or a therapist, you're only a phone call away from a pep talk and a reminder that you *can* do this. At this point, you've learned how to create a psychological, spiritual, medical, and social support system. If you're still not sure if your network is strong enough, consider revisiting the information in chapters 4, 5, and 6.

I'll admit that most of these fears are about situations that are small in the grand scheme of your life with a chronic illness. I certainly have had times that I had to push all this preparedness aside due to a real emergency that no amount of planning would have prevented. What happens if you need to handle serious emergencies on your own?

Managing Medical Emergencies Independently

I've ended up in the emergency room alone, and I won't lie to you and say it isn't a scary place to be. When you're in crisis and you're the only one that can speak on your behalf, the importance of independence loses its appeal. One way I help myself through this is by making sure I've got the important stuff written down. If you do a little planning like this, something as scary and unfamiliar as a lonely ER room is easier to navigate on your own.

I carry a list of current medications, allergies, and a list of past surgeries on a set of laminated notecards in my purse. Just in case

I can't speak for myself, that information will be very clear. Download, photocopy, and fill out the handy online "Medication List Card" and "Emergency List Card" at http://www.newharbinger.com/35999. I also have my emergency contacts listed in my phone under "favorites." This makes it easier for you to find your emergency phone numbers if you're under the haze of medication. You may also want to keep a list of a few different cab companies if you don't have a ridesharing service in your town. Here are a few more things to prepare so that your worst fear doesn't become your worst nightmare:

Setting Yourself Up for Success

Prep #1: Location, Location, Location

You know when it's a great time to live an hour and a half away from your medical team? Never. Save yourself the agony of schlepping down the highway during your worst symptoms. Even if you see your main specialists out of town, set up a local crew of doctors who are going to be able to help you manage the day-to-day care. Same rules apply for your pharmacy, grocery store, at least one or two pizza delivery places, and a gas station. In the face of being stranded from the resources you'll need, making these connections locally or moving to a better location may ultimately be more of a help than a hassle.

Prep #2: Have Your Doctor's Information on Hand

If you're under the care of a regular specialist or general physician, they may be able to guide your ER doctors through your medical history on the phone. If your doctor has a large practice, it may still be difficult to get medical advice when they don't have their file in front of you. Because of this, many patients seek out the help of concierge doctors who often take on smaller patient loads and can more readily recall details from different cases. Generally, contracts with concierge doctors state that they will help guide your care in emergency situations and hospitalizations.

Prep #3: If Possible, Bring a Body

Even if your mom, husband, best friend, brother, or nana can't make it to the ER with you, try as hard as you possibly can to get a friend (of any caliber) to at least help you get checked in. Sometimes just having a familiar face in the room to hurry up the doctor when you're bleeding out of your eyeballs can be useful.

Prep #4: Remember Your Nurse's Name and Ask for a Call Button

This is a critical detail. Remembering your nurse's name insures liability. While you're in the ER, the nurse should know you're not only going to remember her name and the fact that she likes cartoons on her scrubs, but also that if she doesn't wash her hands before handling your port, she is going to get reported to her supervisor.

Asking for a call button is also key. Once you're down, there's a good possibility that between the IV and heart monitors you may not be able to get back up. Being able to buzz the nurses for assistance can save you a lot of stress (and possibly wet sheets).

What's the Worst That Could Happen?

Fear is just the accumulation of unknowns. An exercise my mother used to do with me was to ask:

"What's the worst that could happen?"

And then I would answer, "I'd be sick in the middle of the night and wouldn't be able to get a ride to the hospital!"

She would ask, "And then what?"

"Well," I'd say, feeling angry that wasn't enough. "Then I'd have no ride to the hospital."

"And then what?"

"Then I'd probably have to call 911 and get an ambulance. Or maybe just a cab."

"And then what?"

"And then I'd…get there eventually, I guess. But it would suck."

It's annoying when someone makes you see reason when you've been clinging to fear to stop yourself from taking risks. This exercise helped me to realize that while the outcomes of my fears weren't always pleasant, they more often than not did not result in my intense suffering. Chances are, your fears have already transpired in one form or another. Challenge your anxiety the next time it creeps up on you. What would happen? And what would you do? Have a plan and worry less.

The Key to Independence: Accept the Unexpected

My life is filled with unknowns. I have very little control over what's going on in my body. I can't stop a migraine if it's coming. I can't control how quickly I'll dehydrate or how a new food will affect my stomach. I've accidently dropped my last pill down the drain more times than I want to admit. A good rule to remember when it comes to outsmarting chronic illness is that you can't prevent situations from happening a hundred percent of the time. But, the preparations and tips provided in this chapter will save you lots of hassle.

Ultimately, you can't prepare for a situation you don't see coming. There will be many instances where you'll have to just cock your head to the side and say, "Huh. I did not know that cannoli was going to make an attempt on my life," before ducking into the nearest convenient store bathroom with the most profound regret.

At some point, you will look at your choices and think: *I knew better. I may have wanted a different outcome, but I knew better.* You need to start balancing your risks and benefits. For example, *If I decide to go shopping this afternoon, will I have enough energy to go to the movies tonight? I really want dessert, but my stomach is already a seven on the flare scale. Will a slice of cake throw me over the edge?*

Independence will mean being accountable for any and every way you decide to tip the scales. There will come a point where you can't push yourself, you can't make everyone happy, you can't pay all the bills, and you can't be there for every person in your life. The question to ask yourself is, who and what gets priority?

What Is Your Priority?

Moving out was a huge boost to my self-esteem and it will be the same for you. Knowing that I could survive on my own was extremely gratifying. It gave me hope about the direction of my life. It was high up on my list of priorities. For me to remain independent, I had to be able to afford it, which meant that I had to be able to work. For me to be able to handle all my clients, I had to be constantly on top of my health.

Hospitalizations meant unpaid leave. I couldn't avoid all of them, but I needed to do everything in my power to make them as short and as infrequent as possible. Having a solid treatment plan and a doctor who was available to help me make medication choices was a must. I also realized that I needed to act preventatively. That meant making sure I was at my doctor at the same time every week to get IVs. It also meant starting an exercise regimen through a cardiac rehab program at the hospital to keep up my strength. I also had to stay on top of my medication refills.

Frankly, being sick gave me near-heroic powers of organization. It completely transformed the way I looked at different parts of my life. For example, how important was it really that I made a home-made soufflé every holiday when it almost always cost me as much energy as I would need to attend the dinner? If scrubbing my apartment floor was going to knock me out of commission for two days, wasn't it financially more responsible to hire a housekeeper?

I did a serious intake of what really mattered to me. For me, it is spending time with my family and friends and my dog. It is about focusing on my career so I can have a good quality of life. I didn't need to keep up with everyone I went to high school with and aggressively stalked online. I didn't need to cook dinner for my fiancé every night. I didn't need to put on the song and dance for my in-laws, my judgmental relatives, or even my nosey professors or coworkers. All I needed to do was take care of my needs, and make sure my bills were paid and my health was stable.

What do you feel is your most important priority in service of your independence? Is it focusing fully on your career or school and pushing your schedule to the limit? Is it stabilizing your treatment by experimenting with newer drugs and therapies that might have unknown side-effects? Is it training a new puppy or nurturing a new relationship? Whatever your priority, hopefully the tools in this chapter will help you to plan and create safeguards for a more autonomous life with chronic illness.

CHAPTER 9

Becoming Your Own Patient Advocate

It is your body and your responsibility to treat it with confidence, intelligence, and above all, compassion. You need to own every nerve ending, every cell, and every action you take using this body of yours. You should never let anyone take away your right to make the choices you believe are best for it. Being your own patient advocate means fighting for your opinions about your treatment to be heard. Have you been using your voice? Have you been heard?

Often, when the prescription pad is pulled out of the doctor's pocket, most patients don't interject. Why would you? You're not the doctor here! Maybe you agree that the medication will work best for you if your doctor says so. Maybe you have no idea what kind of fungus is growing on your foot, and you trust your doctor to give you the right ointment. However, you must know that there is a significant difference between being blindly led into the wilds of unknown treatment, and being consciously guided by someone you feel is qualified to have an opportunity to earn your trust.

Smart patients understand that their treatment is a collaborative effort. It takes both the educated patient and the educated physician to find, test, and maintain good health. Being an advocate for yourself doesn't mean recklessly shooting down every medical opinion you don't agree with and it certainly doesn't mean changing your course of treatment without a consult with your doctor.

Being your own advocate means:

- Recognizing the weight of your choices

- Doing the background research on doctors and choosing the best medical ally

- Maximizing the amount of time you have with your doctor by being clear, composed, and knowledgeable about your medical history

- Knowing when to change your medical care team

- Being a proactive patient

- Fighting for your quality of life

It's no question that being your own advocate is a lot of work. Suddenly, you've gone from being a bystander to an active participant in your care. You're now doing the research, asking the major questions, and finding the confidence to speak up. If you want the most out of life with chronic illness, you're going to have to fight for it.

The Choices You'll Make

From my first fight with my pediatrician over antibiotics to my insistence that fiber would be a poor addition to my diet with gastroparesis, I've had many all-out fights with gastroenterologists and nutritionists who have recommended different diets without taking a strong look at my disease and its symptoms. It's been up to me to educate my physicians and if they refuse to be educated, I've often had to refuse their care. There are only so many times you can eat a kale salad before you fully succumb to the idea that your stomach finds it indigestible.

It can be a world of protest for patients with chronic, invisible, progressive, and life-long diseases, whose long-term treatment can mean switching on and off medications and trying new or off-label scripts. Doctors, nurses, and insurance companies can sometimes be barriers against your medical opportunities. Take their advice with a grain of salt because even though they really do want what's best for you, they don't always know what that is.

You can't be afraid to speak up, argue, or worry that you're being cumbersome with your line of questioning. Somebody's got to make the judgment call and when it's your quality of life on the line, you'll find that you will be that annoying, overly analytical patient. When you hit the wall of your doctor's tolerance you may feel like you've overstepped. When you feel guilty about it, dig deep and tell yourself to get over it. This isn't an oil change on your car. This is the only body you're going to have your whole life. Its wellbeing comes before good manners. You have spent your whole life coming to terms with what you can't change. These medical interventions are a key place for you to exercise your free will and shape your life.

The older I get, the more I know with real certainty that no one knows best—not your mom, doctor, best friend, or that guy online. Nobody has the table of contents. This is a "choose your own adventure" kind of story. You make the final decision on what medications you take, what surgeries you go through, whose hands you put yourself in, and most importantly, whose voice you choose to speak for you when you cannot speak for yourself.

Finding a Medical Ally

While it may not seem like a huge hurtle for others, managing your healthcare when you have an active disease is a large responsibility. Selecting your own doctors, researching your own medications and surgeries, handling your health insurance, and monitoring your stress and mental health is a full-time job. Even though you may be able to delegate some medical responsibilities to the doctors you feel are competent, you must always take the lead. This doesn't mean arguing against every suggested medical opinion, it just means making sure that the professionals around you are on the same page as you.

How can you ensure that you and your medical team are on the same page? Discuss your thoughts and opinions before the appointment and do your research. Being a prepared patient helps your team to focus in on the best solutions. My goals vary from specialist to specialist. When it comes to my ENT doctor, I want to make sure he gets the right cultures for any infection I might have. I've discussed my immune deficiency disease with him, and it's important to me that I only ever go on antibiotics when they're one hundred percent necessary and when we've tested a culture to see what it is resistant to. Because of this communication, I can avoid multiple prescriptions for the wrong problem! By sticking to my guns and making sure my wishes are followed through on, I've managed to make a positive impact on my care.

Finding a New Doctor When You're Undiagnosed

When you're still searching for a diagnosis, it's important to find a doctor who has the time and capabilities to do the necessary testing and research you'll need. How can you know who has the time when you're flipping through your insurance booklet? Or worse, how do you find a good match when you have no insurance and have limited options of where you can be treated?

First thing you'll need to do is consult with a primary care physician (PCP), also known as a general internist, so they can categorize your symptoms and push you toward the right specialist. You can find one either through a list you can request from your insurance company or simply by searching online for an internist in your area. Word of mouth and online reviews and ratings can be helpful, but you'll probably get the soundest advice about the doctor through their office manager. When making an appointment, ask their office the following: "I'm an undiagnosed patient with a large cluster of symptoms. I may need to sit with the doctor longer than ten minutes to explain everything. Do you think he has the time to consider this, and if so, what would be the best time of the day to schedule my appointment with him?" You may also want to ask what his patient load is. You'll want to find a doctor with a small patient load if possible. This means they don't have to double book as often and you'll spend less time in the waiting room and more time with the treating physician.

Before you see a general internist, you'll want to call and speak directly to someone at your insurance company. You'll need to ask whether you'll need a referral to see a specialist. You'll also want to ask what the co-pay is to see a specialist and if testing that is done in-office is covered by your co-pay. If you don't have coverage, it's time to consider low-income insurance options in your area.

Finding a New Doctor After a Diagnosis

If you've already been diagnosed, and you're looking for a specialist, you'll be able to narrow down the right physician for you a lot more easily. You'll want to ask the same questions to make sure this doctor has the time and patient load to realistically take on a complicated, chronic illness patient. Once you're at your appointment with the doctor, here are a few questions you can ask:

- Do you regularly treat patients with my disease?

- What sort of treatments are the patients you are treating with my disease receiving?

- Are you current on all the new research? (You may want to bring in any papers on new medications you've researched and may want to try.)

- Do you have same day/next day appointments if I have an emergency?

- Are you affiliated with my local hospital and will you be able to direct my treatment in the emergency room and during a hospital stay?

If you don't have insurance and your specialist has decided that you need treatment, you still have some options on how to obtain that care. Hospitals will generally work with patients who need treatments by putting an "affordable" payment plan in place. Drug companies have also been known to sponsor treatment for patients or provide medications for free or at a discounted price.

Considering a Concierge Doctor

You may be wondering what a concierge doctor is. Maybe you've seen them in movies and TV shows? They also exist in the every-day world to treat patients like you and me! These doctors take on a smaller patient load (generally under 300 patients compared to most general internist practices which have well over 1,000 patients.) For an annual or quarterly fee (around $1,800 to $2,000 per year), you'll have a doctor at your beck and call. Perks to having a concierge doctor on retainer are:

- having their personal cell phone number to reach them at all times

- having a doctor who is familiar with your case even without his file in front of you

- having a lead physician to guide your care in the emergency room

These perks can be a huge relief for patients with pain management problems who are constantly scrutinized, patients with complicated medical histories, or patients with rare diseases who have no experts in their area and need someone committed to researching new and innovative treatments. Contrary to popular belief, care by these doctors isn't only for the wealthy. The average cost of a concierge physician is around just $150 per month. That's less than an average car payment or even the cost of a pastry and a coffee each day. Many concierge patients have found that reliable care by a doctor who knows them well resulted in lower health care costs. As a result, there were fewer emergency room visits and long hospitalizations, less unnecessary or repetitive testing, and more preventative care.

Doctor Recommendations, Referrals, and Bad Reviews

I've got an ENT that I'd talk your ear off about. He's *the* best ENT doctor in Boca Raton. I'm sure my sinuses would be forever sealed without his intervention. Recommendations from friends and fellow patients are always great tools in finding the best doctor for you. You'll also want to remain open-eared when it comes to bad recommendations. I had to get through three bad ENTs to get to the good one. Lastly, if you have no friends or fellow patients who will reveal their favorite doctors, look to your general doctor to get a referral. (This only applies to referrals for specialists. Don't ask your doctor for a doctor who can replace them. They don't like that.)

Check out the following websites to get you started:

- **RateMDs.com:** This site offers information and ratings for millions of doctors and health specialists around the world.

- **Zocdoc.com:** This site helps you find a doctor and book appointments instantly. You can also read reviews of each doctor by different patients.

- **Healthgrades.com:** This site provides information on doctors, specialists, and hospitals close to you.

Referrals

When asking your doctor for a referral to a specialist, you must be very specific about what you're looking for. Doctors may work frequently with just one doctor, so they may suggest just that one doctor that they know. If they can't suggest more than just that one doctor, that's how you know they're picking from a limited pool. Ask questions like, "Why do you recommend him?" You'll want to know if they're recommending them because they're a good doctor or a good friend. Make sure to also ask if the doctor has performed this procedure on a lot of their patients. A doctor can always recommend another doctor for treatment, but make sure he's doing it specifically for the needs of your treatment. Lastly, ask which hospitals the doctor is affiliated with. This is a good question to ask to make sure that if you need to be hospitalized, the doctor will be able to visit you there to direct your care.

Bad Reviews

What if you've heard bad things about a doctor, but you're unsure if they're true or not? While most people would steer clear either way, you may have a limited number of physicians to choose from through your insurance company. Start by doing your own investigative process. Search online for more reviews about the doctor. Call the doctor's front office and ask salient questions about their care. Review their education and experience level. If you're feeling brave, go in for a consultation. Sometimes a short visit is worth the time spent to not miss out on what could be a good physician.

Recommendations

Some people just like to brag about how well connected they are. Just because they know and have seen a thousand doctors doesn't mean that all of them had a great bedside manner and cured cancer during their fifteen-minute consult. When someone gives a good review, make sure to ask specific questions like: "Was the doctor familiar with your disease or did you have to explain it to them? Did they go over your entire medical history or just want the highlights? Did they read up on any new treatments or were they recommending a lot of things you'd already tried?"

Your Recommendations

Don't forget that it's your duty as a patient to keep that flow of information going. If you find a good doctor, shout it from the mountaintops! Don't you wish that someone had steered you clear of that wacko surgeon that botched your surgery or kept you from even entering the geneticist's office at that teaching hospital who made it his mission to humiliate patients in front of his teaching students? Doctors may vow to do no harm, but it is the patients who keep the good ones in business long enough to keep that promise. Now you have the tools to find the right care for you. Let's put them to use.

Ready to Choose?

Found a doctor who might be a good fit, but you're just not *quite* sure yet? You can do your research online or by checking with your referring doctor. Make sure you know and feel comfortable with the answers to the following questions before you decide.

- Is this doctor board certified? Are they licensed? (Check with your state's medical licensing board if this isn't explicitly listed in their credentials.)

- How long have they been practicing?

- Do they have any malpractice suits against them?

- Are they affiliated with your local hospital?

- Do they have malpractice insurance? If not, why?

- Do they take your insurance or can you work out an affordable financing plan for treatment?

- If the doctor you're researching is a surgeon, consider the success rate of their past surgeries. How many have they performed?

Comparing Treatment

Most patients with chronic illness eventually develop a second or third condition. New diseases mean new symptoms, which means new treatments. Researching your new prescriptions can be helpful and it's always smart to do your own research. Connecting with people who have had a similar surgery you're considering or are currently taking a new drug you're about to try can be a valuable source of information. When you pool a patient community's knowledge of treatments, you end up opening doors you and your doctor probably haven't even considered. How you evaluate a new prescription is similar to how you would refer, recommend, and rate a doctor. Ask around, look for reviews from other patients, and ask other patients to share their personal experiences. Did they react with certain symptoms? What has been the long-term outcome of taking this medication? Has it been a financial burden or has the insurance company been gracious about getting the generic? Did it do its job?

The crux of patient advocacy can really be summed up into just that: Did the doctor, hospital, or treatment do its job? Was I treated with respected during it? In the next section, advocate Lauren Stiles talks about incorporating these two points into your basic fifteen-minute doctor exam.

Getting the Most Out of Your 15 Minutes

Stiles is the CEO and co-founder of Dysautonomia International, a patient organization that offers resources, organizes research, and hosts an annual conference for patients. Stiles has served in leadership positions on government councils, non-profit boards, and professional associations. She developed dysautonomia (postural orthostatic tachycardia syndrome) symptoms overnight at age thirty-one. After a relentless two-year quest to find an underlying cause for her symptoms, she was finally diagnosed with autonomic neuropathy caused by an autoimmune disease, Sjogren's syndrome. Since co-founding Dysautonomia International in 2012, Stiles has been an outspoken advocate for individuals living with autonomic disorders. She has lectured on autonomic disorders at the National Institute of Health, Duke University, Harvard University, and Stony Brook University. Her work educating patients on how to receive the best care has hugely impacted the invisible disease community.

If you are lucky enough to find a doctor who spends more than the usual fifteen minutes with you, that's wonderful, but most of us are going to have to deal with those "it's over before you blink" visits from time to time, especially when seeing a new specialist.

You may have waited two years and sold your family heirlooms to get an appointment with Dr. Big Expectations, but you aren't going to have all the time you want to tell him about your 101 weird symptoms, all the tests you've had, all the treatments that didn't work, and why you fired your last idiot doctor.

Assume you have fifteen minutes. You may be given more time, but it's important to have realistic expectations. This is the reality of the hamster treadmill that is modern medicine. Your doctor is probably not being brief with you because he's a jerk. He just has forty other patients to see that day, several hours of ridiculous forms to fill out, a hundred emails to read and respond to, and seventy phone calls to make before he goes home today. Doctors have the highest suicide rate of any profession because they are so stressed out. So, don't take it personally when you don't get all the time you need. No one else is getting the time they need either, including your doctor.

Before you even make the appointment, ask yourself: "Why do I want to see this doctor?" This should be the goal of your visit. Does she have a special skill that may benefit you? Does he offer a test or treatment that you want to look into? Are you just looking for a second opinion? The following exercise is a great way for patients to get clarity on their needs before heading into an appointment.

Make four lists before your appointment on separate pieces of paper:

(a) questions you need answers to, from most pressing to least pressing;

(b) your current symptoms, from most bothersome to least bothersome;

(c) your prior diagnoses; and

(d) your current meds and drug allergies.

Put the date of the office visit and your name on each page. Give these to the doctor or the nursing staff when you arrive and ask them to put a photocopy of each page in your chart. You'll want a copy on hand too when you speak with the doctor.

When you meet the doctor, offer a handshake, a smile, and a "nice to meet you." Doctors are human beings and most of them prefer dealing with friendly patients. You want this doctor to want to help you. As chronic illness patients, we have probably seen our fair share of crappy doctors that leave us feeling frustrated and angry. Don't hold this against your new doctor. Assume he or she will be fabulous, until proven otherwise.

Doctors usually begin the appointment by asking what's wrong. This is when you tell them the goal of your visit. Use phrases like, "I'm hoping you can…" or "I would like your help in finding out…." Don't give orders like, "I need you to…" or "I want you to…." Be deferential to the doctor, without being a pushover or a kiss up. Be focused and rely on your written questions during the appointment. Don't say bad things about other doctors or hospitals, even if they were total jerks.

Whatever you do, don't bring a giant binder of medical records into the exam room! If you are a chronic illness patient, you probably have a forest worth of trees in paperwork on your prior lab results, doctor's notes, imaging studies, etc. It's fine to bring this to your appointment, but you will scare off most doctors if this is the first impression they have of you. Leave the binder in the car or with a friend in the waiting room. If you need to bring it in to the exam room, put it in a backpack so it doesn't become the elephant in the room as you try to have a focused conversation with your doctor. That binder can very easily be misinterpreted as hypochondriac, attention seeker, or patient that is too complicated to get involved with. If the doctor wants any of your prior medical records, you can find out what they want, and give the relevant documents to their secretary after the appointment to make copies of, or you can offer to fax it to them after your visit.

As you end your visit, make sure you understand the game plan moving forward. Is the doctor ordering tests or writing a prescription? Where do you go for the tests? Who will get the insurance approval for the tests? How will you get the results? When should you come back for a follow-up?

Don't forget to end your visit with a "thanks for your time." Grandma's advice comes to mind: "You get more bees with honey."

When is it Time to Change Your Health Care Team?

When my medication fails time after time, the emergency room visits become too close together, and my assigned diet is not working, I wonder: Is it time to find a new doctor? Sometimes doctors can get complacent with our care. We'll have a short discussion about some new symptoms, but overall there are no major changes suggested in terms of new medications or therapies. No new testing is done, and you begin to get the idea that your doctor is very plainly saying, "Well, this is as good as it's going to get, kid!" If you find yourself in that situation and you feel you cannot convince your doctor to find new solutions to your care, take that as a clear sign to find another physician who might know of another option.

Deciding when to make a change in your health care is a constant in self-advocacy. It's important to do a serious evaluation from time-to-time to see if your needs are really being met by your doctor. You should always be evaluating your quality of life and demanding the best out of it. Your doctor should be on your team, in your court, and with their head fully in the game. How do you know if your current doctor is the right one for you?

Start by asking yourself these questions:

- Do I feel like my symptoms are under control?

- Are my questions being answered in a way I can understand?

- Am I getting back full reports on my blood tests and other diagnostics?

- Do I feel comfortable with the medications I'm on or do I think we could do better?

- Does my doctor have enough time for me? Are my appointments being cut short or being rushed?

- Is my doctor available to me during emergencies?

- Is my treatment in the ER being managed by them? Are they or someone else in their office familiar with my condition available by phone or email in case of emergencies?

If you're answering "no" or "not really" to most of these questions, then it's probably time to start looking for a new doctor.

For me, and many other patients with complicated diseases, needing to find a new health care team after a few years is something that happens without fail. I've had three main quarterbacks for my medical team in the past five years. While I can say with confidence that each doctor was capable, qualified, and worked hard to help me manage my disease, they ultimately reached a point where they could no longer offer insight on what would be my next step. My disease is progressive; it was only natural that I had to move on from my team and transition to a new set of professionals who would be able to take on the next round of research with fresh eyes.

It's okay to say that you need to move on from a team, even if the doctors have become an essential part of your treatment. It comes down to your quality of life and whether it's getting worse, better, or staying the same. Quality of life should always be improving. If your doctor can no longer figure out how to bring your care to the next level, it's time to let them go.

Letting Someone Else Advocate for You

There have been far too many moments where I've sat face to face with my doctor, having just received instructions from them, and all I can do is look at them and say, "Huh?" Painkillers. Exhaustion. Brain fog. We won't always be able to put our best foot forward as a patient advocate when the patient we are trying to advocate for is ourselves. Before you find yourself in a bind, it's good to designate a person in your support tribe and ask for their help. This person can be a friend, a parent, a relative, a nurse aid. And if you're completely alone, there is technology and tools to help you stay afloat. (Hold tight, we'll talk about that in a minute.)

What are the qualities you'll want to look for in a potential advocate? Well, that's kind of like saying you'd like to pre-select the nicest seat on the public bus you're taking tomorrow. You most likely will not get to choose who will take you to appointments and help you through them. You'll get whoever volunteers and you'll say thank you with a smile on your face even if you can't stand them. They don't need a medical degree, or need to know your entire medical history. They just need to be able to take notes, ask questions on your behalf, and work to not make you feel like you've put an unfortunate dent in their day's schedule. The last thing you need during the whirlwind of disorientation is a guilt trip for being a burden.

At this point in my life, I wouldn't say that I'm necessarily "scared" to go to the doctor. I've been subjected to some pretty awful (yet, very common) tests and my fears of shots, scopes, and speculums are just about gone. There is still one thing that brings me uneasiness when going to see a new doctor. I fear that they will reject my case, citing that it's too complicated or that they won't have the time.

During a very bad flare-up where I was floating between internists, I asked my husband to accompany me to a new doctor. My husband was a great source of comfort for me as we waited in the office for the doctor to finish up with another patient. The appointment, for the most part, went very well. The doctor understood my disease and was very empathetic and had great suggestions. However, at the very end of the meeting he said he was sorry, but that he couldn't take me on as a patient. He just didn't have the time for such a complicated case.

I was crushed. We had been waiting for this appointment for weeks and in the meantime I was spread thin trying to keep a lid on my out-of-control symptoms. In the car on the way home my husband turned to me and said he was sorry it hadn't worked out.

He also made me remember that the doctor said he would talk to the two other physicians in his office, and that one of them would surely be able to take me on while he was in and out of the country for a family emergency.

"It's going to all work out," my husband said, having no way of knowing this for sure. "We'll meet with the other doctors and if we need to, we'll keep meeting with other doctors. We'll find someone."

It was exactly what I needed to hear at exactly the right time. It was something I would have told myself if I was alone in the car on my way home from this appointment. But having somebody else say it to me first made a world of difference in how I looked at the situation. I thanked him for telling me that and for taking me to the appointment. He brushed it off, but the truth is that if he weren't with me, this would have been a long and tearful ride home.

Get over your humiliation of being carted around. Get over your concern that you're putting people out by asking them for their help. Get over yourself because pride is a much easier pill to swallow than the reality of what happens when you don't put your healthcare as your priority. You are where you are, and you're going to have to make the best of it. Part of that is helping others feel as useful as possible in a situation where they also feel powerless. Remember, this is a key part of improving the understanding of your disease between you and your network of loved ones. Give them an opportunity to assist you. Here are some things you can do help your advocate help you.

- Say, "Thank you, that was really kind of you to take time out of your schedule to help me get through my appointment."

- Ask them to help you remember questions or concerns you want to bring up but might forget about once you enter the exam room.

- Give them a piece of paper and a pen and ask them to record some of the information from the doctor's appointment so you can read it later.

- Let them ask their questions too. They may not have a say in what treatment path you ultimately choose, but one more person in the trenches with you who has all the information is always an asset.

Start thinking about selecting the appropriate people in your life to advocate for you when you cannot do so for yourself. There is only one real requirement for someone being your advocate: They should give a crap about you!

Being a Proactive Patient

Don't you just want to burn every health magazine and pamphlet that has the phrase, "Be a proactive patient" on it? It's like, "Oh, I'm sorry. I didn't know you're not supposed to walk on glass or eat gas station sushi!" Of course, I'm being proactive. I'm not *actively* being *negligent* of my health. As much as the phrase irks me, I've made it my mission to redefine it from its nasty stigmatization and into something that makes sense. I want to be a proactive patient. I want to do my personal best to make sure my body makes the most of its core defenses. Below is a list of ways in which you can be that kind of "proactive patient."

- Fight to remain conscious when you are in the middle of doctor's appointments.

- Eat as close to a healthy diet as your condition will allow. Try to not give into the urge to eat cheat foods that may cause a flare-up.

- Make sure to exercise regularly, even if that means doing laps around your hospital floor during an inpatient stay.

- Stay on top of your payment plans for medical bills.

- Be happy. When you feel well, see your friends, go to a party, have a night out, go on a date, see a new movie, or just lay outside in the grass and appreciate the sweet smell of not being in the emergency room.

Being proactive is about being responsible for your own happiness, but it also means being responsible for your weaker moments, as we discussed in chapter 8. Remember that preparation is your best friend when you are at your most vulnerable and your head is cloudy. When a serious issue needs to be resolved during a doctor or hospital visit, here are a few ways to keep you one step ahead of the brain fog:

- Have a list of your personal information, including your full name, date of birth, address, contact person, and address.

- Have a list of the medications you are currently on. Update this list as regimens change.

- Have a list of your allergies to medications.

- Get a medical identification bracelet.

- If you think you won't be able to remember the doctor's instructions, ask them if it would be okay to record your consult on your phone, or if they can speak slowly so you can write things down on a notepad.

True Advocacy: Valuing Your Quality of Life

It all comes down to these three words: quality of life. That's not just a phrase reserved for those on their deathbed, struggling to decide whether they should continue their treatment. It's a phrase for all patients in all situations and I make sure to keep it lit up in the back of my mind for even my most trivial medical choices. Sometimes it's as simple as deciding that your quality of life would be improved if you didn't have to take the highway to get to your internist's inconvenient office. But many times, it comes down to decisions like: Will the quality of my life change if this medication that improves my blood pressure also reduces my libido? Or will my overall quality of life be improved if I decide to have this surgery, even if it puts me out of commission in the short term?

Many patients forget to make their quality of life a priority when they face a long road of chronic illness. They feel undeserving of a quality life because of the inconvenience and disappointment their disease might inflict on the lives of those they love. Sometimes their doctors don't offer choices, and they just decide to be treated by the book instead of asking for alternatives and seeking second opinions. There are many reasons doctors treat patients by the book. It's important to remember that *you* are the ultimate deciding factor in your treatment. You have a right to refuse treatment you feel will not be worth the benefit. You have a right to seek out another opinion by another physician. You can say, "That isn't good enough."

When facing choices that affect your quality of life, ask yourself these questions:

- Will it alter my appearance and disrupt my self-esteem?

- Will it reduce my ability to enjoy good food, entertainment, or company with my friends?

- Will it mean I'll have to stop working and rely on someone or something else for financial support?

- Will it give me anxiety each time I need to deal with it?

- Does it make me depressed every time I think about it?

- Will it cause more pain than I'm equipped to deal with?

- What are my alternatives?

For me, it was important to test different medications to see if they could improve my condition. If I found out that they couldn't help me and that major lifestyle changes were the only way to a better quality of life, it made it easier for me to accept and commit to those lifestyle changes.

Over the course of your illness, you'll experiment with medications, change doctors, switch hospitals, have surgeries, adjust your diet and exercise regimen, and experience different sleep patterns. You will make mistakes, regret decisions you've made, and wish you had done things better or smarter. But it's important not to view these blips in judgment as mistakes, but as opportunities to ask yourself questions like the following:

- What am I willing to give up to feel my best?

- What side effects am I willing to put up with?

- How much time and energy do I want to commit to treatments?

- How much suffering am I willing to endure?

- What doctors do I trust?

- What specialists are most knowledgeable about my disease?

- How can I communicate my symptoms most effectively?

- What preventative steps can I take to give myself the best chance of overcoming disease flare-ups?

These questions allow you to take a step back in the middle of medical chaos and examine whether you're going in the right direction and remind yourself of what you want out of life. Are you comfortable with the way you're being cared for? Have you been pushed in a direction you weren't comfortable with? You always have the option of taking control and addressing the issues of living well with a life-limiting disease. You are deserving of living a life with dignity, honesty, and direction. So, demand it!

CHAPTER 10

Thriving with Chronic Illness

When I first started my blog, I decided to name it "Let's Feel Better." I thought that was what I wanted. Isn't that what all patients want? To feel better? As I went through this great adventure of learning to live with a chronic disease, I did find my better days. They came when I had better doctors, better treatments, and better medication. Better was a concept that I ached for. I thought if my health got better, I would be happy again—my stress would decrease, I would be more independent, and I would have more opportunities in relationships and career. I did eventually get to a point where I was better. And I learned that *better is not enough.*

You will face mountains and molehills through the trials of your disease. You'll pick your battles, stand your ground, and accept things you couldn't have imagined accepting when you were healthier. Your doctors will tell you at some point that your symptoms have improved. Your treatments will keep things at their status quo. You will be told that *you are a survivor.* But, surviving a chronic illness is not enough.

Much of this book has been about learning to accept the limitations of your disease, finding joy in your new reality, and giving yourself the chance to excel in a way that best supports your health. What I hope you've also come to understand is that you deserve to thrive, to seek your ultimate happiness, and to not believe that feeling better than you did yesterday is enough.

Thriving with a chronic illness is an ongoing journey. When you have accepted your disease, learned to adjust your life around it, and reorganized your plans and goals, the next step is not just to feel better but to feel your very best and believe that you deserve to have the best doctors, the best treatment, and the most supportive people in your life as you move forward.

Are you only better? Or are you at your best? This chapter will help you access where you're at. Will you be living in the moment or letting the stress of your disease sweep away your attention? Are you giving yourself the voice you need to power through the condemnation, pity, and judgments of others? Are you in a place where you're making your treatment choices not just based on what will hit the hardest but also on what will give your life the greatest quality?

Live in the Moment

Have you ever been on a romantic date but had something else on your mind? Maybe you worried about your kids at home with the sitter or were waiting on an important response from work. Instead of focusing on the good food and excellent company, you couldn't stop staring at your cell phone. While most people are familiar with these small interruptions, those with chronic illness are constantly distracted by their body's messages or by the fear that their body has a rude message to send soon. Is the dinner choice going to affect your stomach? Will it ruin your plans for later? Will fatigue sneak in during time with friends, forcing you to end the night early? Could brain fog make conversing difficult? Will a symptom need to be explained before you're ready to speak about it?

It's a struggle to live fully in the moment without wondering: What new symptom will knock me down next? When you've started to use the tools in this book to begin managing the chaos of your disease, you'll be in a place where you can start to choose where you want to be. Do you want to be here at the table, talking to the person in front of you? Or do you want to be thinking about how to talk to your boss about why you had to cancel another important meeting for a more important doctor appointment? You will be able to give yourself permission to say: I am allowed to be here now. I can have this life no matter how hopeless each interruption may have seemed in the past. Yes, your disease will take up its own roomy space in your mind, but you can have a life that exists outside of your illness. Begin to visualize your disease and all its "what ifs" as a wet umbrella. Whenever you walk into the room of each new moment, envision yourself taking that umbrella and leaving it by the door.

Focus on Your Quality of Life, Not Your Diagnosis

When a disease is hard to diagnose, we can spend years trying to find the answer to questions like: "Is it because of a parasite? Bacteria? A cancer?" There is an infinite list of possibilities as to why you could be sick. But after a while, you've got to take a break from the endless hunt for answers and ask yourself, "How am I going to handle living with my disease today?"

You don't want your life to just be about going from doctor to doctor. You need balance—time to spend with friends and family and to do the things that really matter to you. You can't hunt, search, question, or get an answer for any of the whys in life until you've mastered feeding yourself, moving yourself, and balancing your work, relationships, and symptoms at the same time. If you don't take the time to do those things, you aren't really living. Whether you've been diagnosed, are in treatment, or are still struggling to put a name to the disease that is haunting you, you need to find acceptance. It's not defeat. It's not giving up. It's learning how to continue growing, striving, and thriving even when chronic illness stands resolutely in your way. Maybe in the past you've felt like the victim, but now you have some tools to reclaim your life.

Advocate for Yourself

At the time when I was being told by many doctors that I was faking my illness, I couldn't imagine a reality where I'd be able to stand up for myself. My disease is, in every respect, my responsibility. Fighting for a better quality of life is a constant. You need to wake up each morning and ask yourself, "How can my life be improved?"

When you're advocating for yourself, it means you're empowering yourself through information and education. You're doing your research and fulfilling your duty as the owner of your body to know—not to be told—what options you have. This information can be found through your knowledgeable physicians, but it can also be explored in books, online, through a disease-related organization, and most importantly, in discussion with other patients! This book has shown you multiple ways in which you can reach out to get the latest information to best benefit you throughout your treatment. Once you have your options, the next step is weighing them carefully. You'll want to discuss them at length with your doctor, partner, friends, or family. If you're too scared to ask your questions and demand the answers you deserve, you may find yourself disappointed by your doctor and their treatment plan.

Misinformation and misunderstanding can result in shame, which is what leads patients to stop themselves from taking action, both medically and therapeutically. So, please don't be scared to share the fruits of your research and the value of your personal experience with other patients through support groups and websites. Do your part by joining in on the conversation. Ultimately, how you choose to handle your disease will dictate how you experience your life. Only you can determine what will give you the greatest freedom. Only you can define what "truly living" with your chronic illness feels like to you.

Stay One Step Ahead

Remember when we talked about preparing for a tsunami instead of a rainy day? You should feel plenty prepared now! I can practically hear the squeak of your boots and the drops on your umbrella. Money? Made and saved. ER plans? The address is already plugged into your GPS. Fallen on the floor and panicked you won't be able to get back up? Nope, because you're one step ahead of whatever your disease is going to throw at you. If you are still unsure, go back to chapter 8 to review how to establish the groundwork for autonomy in your adult life.

Outsmart Your Disease and Don't Forget to Plan for Your Happiness

Managing chronic illness means developing strategies to assist you in moving forward with your life's greater focus, and with as minimal suffering as possible. Don't head-butt your disease, outsmart it. Outsmart it in your relationships by breaking down those silent barriers with the hard questions: "Is this too much for you?" "Do you resent me?" "Do you believe this is a real condition, with symptoms worthy of the extremes I'm using to treat them?" Outsmart it by making plans of action to create that greater net of support and to give your friends, family and partners the information they need to understand what you're experiencing and how they can help. Outsmart it in your classroom, your workplace, your doctor's office, and at the family dinner table. Outsmart it when you feel like you can't find your way around the endless monstrosity of it. Outsmart it because you *feel* and you *know* that you deserve all the privileges and opportunities that others have.

In this book, you've learned how to evaluate your living situation to see if you are ready to go out on your own, and how you can make the process safe and comfortable. You've also learned how to address your needs at school or work and maximize your flexibility when other people are needing things from you. With these safeguards in place, there is plenty of room to be the person your illness may have prevented you from becoming. With all the planning we've discussed so far, the one thing you don't want to forget is to plan for is your happiness. Yes, you will have to make adjustments to create a functioning life, but it can and should also be ultimately fulfilling.

Continue to Learn and Practice Coping Mechanisms

The world is not going to stop setting you up to fail, sometimes in spectacular fashion. No matter how smart you plan, or how savvy your psychic abilities are, life will throw stuff at you that you didn't see coming. Beyond accepting it, the key to thriving is the way in which you treat yourself and give yourself compassion. In Dawn's words, "Love can heal your pain—the love you actively express towards yourself. The mind and body are intrinsically linked. Love and kindness in your thoughts will improve the health of your body."

There are portions of this book dedicated to establishing a support network, but the truth is, you must be your greatest cheerleader. You must be in charge of going easy on yourself, quieting that inner critic, and loving you for everything that you are. It is easier said than done, but the more we take the time to monitor how we think about ourselves, take time for the comforts we enjoy, and pat ourselves on the back for the superhuman amount of resilience we are capable of, the closer we get to total thriving.

Accept Your Disease

As I've mentioned many times in this book, the main trait a successful, functional patient has is the ability to accept—again and again—whatever comes. As you forge ahead, remember that acceptance has never been the road to giving up. It's just a new perspective, one that you'll find eliminates so much of your inner turmoil. While you may have looked around yourself before and seen a world full of people more capable or strong-willed than you, with acceptance, hopefully you can now see that you too can tap into a deep well of strength and willpower.

Become Your Most Empowered Self

Hopefully this book has opened a new world to you—one where the road ahead to changing your life is much clearer and accessible. If nothing else, I want you to understand that you're more capable of thriving now than you ever have been before. In fact, many with chronic illnesses find that other obstacles in life become laughably trivial after they've started learning to cope with their disease. Deadlines? Bills? Social squabbles? Please. While others struggle with these issues, your perspective from simply trying to keep your head afloat allows you to see what is most important in life. It is a power very few possess. Now is the time to become your most empowered self.

Remember who you are. You've had tubes in places there should never be tubes. You've had bandages ripped off the places you wouldn't wax on your bravest of days. You've had a *reasonable* conversation with your health insurance provider.

I'm not saying you're a superhero or anything.

But...

like...

you're a superhero.

Acknowledgments

Thanks to the many patients who spoke out and shared their story. Thank you to Dawn Wiggins and Kait Scalisi for their invaluable advice. A huge thanks to my mother, husband, friends, family, and those who have been a powerful network of support. And last, but not least, a big thanks to my editors at New Harbinger Publications, Ryan Buresh, Caleb Beckwith, Clancy Drake, and Erin Raber, and my agent Jill Marsal for helping to make this book a reality.

Appendix: Online Resources

General Resources

The American Autoimmune Related Diseases Association

http://www.aarda.org

The American Autoimmune Related Diseases Association is dedicated to the eradication of autoimmune diseases and the alleviation of the socioeconomic impact of autoimmunity. They accomplish this through facilitating collaboration in the areas of education, public awareness, research, and patient services in an effective, ethical, and efficient manner.

American Gastroenterology Association

http://www.gastro.org

Founded in 1897, the AGA has grown to include more than 16,000 members from around the globe who are involved in all aspects of the science, practice, and advancement of gastroenterology. The AGA, a 501(c6) organization, administers all membership and public policy activities, while the AGA Institute, a 501(c3) organization, runs the organization's practice, research, and educational programs.

American Thyroid Association

http://www.thyroid.org

The ATA is the leading organization devoted to thyroid biology and to the prevention and treatment of thyroid disease through excellence in research, clinical care, education, and public health.

The Arthritis Foundation

http://www.arthritis.org

The Arthritis Foundation is the largest national nonprofit organization that supports more than a hundred types of arthritis and related conditions. The foundation offers information and tools to help people live a better life with arthritis, such as advice from medical experts, specialized arthritis self-management, or exercise classes. For every dollar donated to The Arthritis Foundation, seventy-eight cents goes directly to fund research and activities for people with arthritis.

Celiac Disease Foundation

http://celiac.org

CDF has played a crucial role in improving the lives of those afflicted with celiac disease. They sponsored the first serology workshop (which led to today's celiac disease blood test), advocated on Capitol Hill for gluten-free labeling laws, partnered with mainstream manufacturers to create today's gluten-free marketplace, and offered the number one website for celiac disease. With a range of vital programs and services for the public, patients, healthcare professionals, and food industries, CDF meets the growing public health challenge of diagnosing and treating celiac disease and other gluten-related disorders.

Chronic Connect

http://www.chronicconnect.org

Chronic Connect Incorporated seeks to serve the chronic illness community by providing resources and community for patients. It develops technology that allows patients to find local support, sending care packages to both patients and caregivers in need, and creating programs for patient and caregiver support and education.

The Crohn's and Colitis Foundation of America (CCFA)

http://www.ccfa.org

Founded in 1967, CCFA has remained at the forefront of research in Crohn's disease and ulcerative colitis. Today, they fund cutting-edge studies at major medical institutions, nurture investigators at the early stages of their careers, and finance underdeveloped areas of research. In addition, their educational workshops and programs, along with their scientific journal, *Inflammatory Bowel Diseases*, enable medical professionals to keep up with this rapidly growing field.

Dysautonomia International

www.dysautonomiainternational.com

This 501(c)(3) non-profit was founded in 2012 by patients, caregivers, physicians, and researchers dedicated to assisting people living with various forms of dysautonomia.

Endometriosis Foundation of America

http://www.endofound.org

The Endometriosis Foundation of America strives to increase disease recognition, provide advocacy, facilitate expert surgical training, and fund landmark endometriosis research. Engaged in a robust campaign to inform both the medical community and the public, the EFA places emphasis on the critical importance of early diagnosis and effective intervention while simultaneously providing education to the next generation of medical professionals and their patients.

Global Genes™

www.globalgenes.org

Global Genes™ is one of the leading rare disease patient advocacy organizations in the world. The non-profit organization promotes the needs of the rare disease community under a unifying symbol of hope—the Blue Denim Genes Ribbon™. What began as a grassroots movement in 2009, with just a few rare disease parent advocates and foundations, is now more than 500 global organizations. Their mission is to eliminate the challenges of rare disease by building awareness and providing critical connections and resources to positively impact affected patients and families.

G-PACT

http://www.g-pact.org

G-PACT provides assistance to patients and families affected by gastroparesis and intestinal pseudo-obstruction in order to improve quality of life and decrease fears surrounding the conditions. Their aim is to provide hope to those who have lost it, support to those who need it, and knowledge to those who do not understand this condition.

IG Living Magazine

http://www.igliving.com

The IG Living magazine's mission is to support the IG community through education, communication, and advocacy. IG Living is the only magazine dedicated to patients who use immune globulin products.

Immune Deficiency Foundation

http://primaryimmune.org

Founded in 1980, the Immune Deficiency Foundation (IDF) is the national non-profit patient organization dedicated to improving the diagnosis, treatment, and quality of life for people with PI through advocacy, education, and research.

International Foundation for Functional Gastrointestinal Disorders

http://www.iffgd.org

The International Foundation for Functional Gastrointestinal Disorders (IFFGD) is a nonprofit education and research organization. Their mission is to inform, assist, and support people affected by gastrointestinal disorders.

Invisible Disabilities Association

https://invisibledisabilities.org

The Invisible Disabilities® Association is passionate about providing awareness that invisible illness, pain, and disabilities are very real. Their mission is to encourage, educate, and connect people and organizations touched by illness, pain, and disability around the globe.

Let's Feel Better

https://www.letsfeelbetter.com

Author Ilana Jacqueline's award-winning blog offers hilarious and heartfelt experiences about coping with chronic illness. From full contact fights with skull-cramping migraines to making peace with being a human pincushion, she writes boldly and unabashedly about breaking down, getting back up, and pulling off the bandage that is "coming out" about the shame and frustration of living with chronic illness.

Lupus Foundation of America

http://www.lupus.org

The Lupus Foundation of America is devoted to solving the mystery of lupus, while giving caring support to those who suffer from its brutal impact. Their mission is to improve the quality of life for all people affected by lupus through programs of research, education, support, and advocacy.

The National Adrenal Diseases Foundation

http://www.nadf.us

The National Adrenal Diseases Foundation informs, educates, and supports those with adrenal disease and their families. Their mission includes stopping unnecessary death from undiagnosed Addison's disease and to improve the quality of life for those living with it.

The National Fibromyalgia Association

http://www.fmaware.org

The National Fibromyalgia Association is a non-profit organization whose mission is to develop and execute programs dedicated to improving the quality of life for people with fibromyalgia.

National Foundation for Celiac Awareness

http://www.celiaccentral.org

Through empowerment, education, advocacy, and research, the National Foundation for Celiac Awareness (NFCA) drives the diagnoses of celiac disease and other gluten-related disorders and improves the quality of life for those on a life-long gluten-free diet. Their goal is to reduce the devastating impact of undiagnosed celiac disease, as well as the contraction of other diseases, such as cancer, diabetes, osteoporosis, and an "autoimmune cascade."

The National Multiple Sclerosis Society

http://www.nationalmssociety.org

The National MS Society mobilizes people and resources to drive research for a cure and to address the challenges of those affected by MS. Headquartered in New York City, this non-profit organization with chapters nationwide helps people affected by MS through funding research, driving change through advocacy, facilitating professional education, and providing programs and services.

The National Organization for Rare Disease (NORD)

https://www.rarediseases.org

The National Organization for Rare Disorders (NORD) is a unique federation of voluntary health organizations dedicated to helping people with rare "orphan" diseases and assisting the organizations that serve them. NORD is committed to the identification, treatment, and cure of rare disorders through programs of education, advocacy, research, and service.

North American Society for Pediatric Gastroenterology, Hepatology, and Nutrition

http://www.naspghan.org

The mission of the North American Society for Pediatric Gastroenterology, Hepatology, and Nutrition is to advance understanding of normal development, physiology, and pathophysiology of diseases of the gastrointestinal tract and liver in children. They also seek to improve quality of care by fostering the dissemination of this knowledge through scientific meetings, professional and public education, and policy development. They serve as an effective voice for members and the profession.

Partnership to Fight Chronic Disease

http://www.fightchronicdisease.org

The Partnership to Fight Chronic Disease (PFCD) is a coalition of hundreds of patient, provider, community, business, labor groups, and health policy experts committed to raising awareness about chronic disease.

Patient Access Network (PAN)

https://panfoundation.org

PAN is an independent non-profit organization that provides assistance to underinsured patients for their out-of-pocket expenses for life-saving medications.

Project Sleep

http://project-sleep.com

Project Sleep is a non-profit organization run by narcolepsy advocate Julie Flygare. Its mission focuses on raising awareness about sleep health and sleep disorders.

Rheumatoid Patient Foundation

http://rheum4us.org

The Rheumatoid Patient Foundation provides a complete understanding of the disease for health professionals and the public. They seek to provide comprehensive education on how rheumatoid will impact patients' relationships, medical care, employment, and health insurance.

Scleroderma Foundation

http://www.scleroderma.org

The Scleroderma Foundation is the national organization for people with scleroderma and their families and friends. Their three-fold mission includes helping to support patients and their families who are coping with this disease through mutual support programs, peer counseling, physician referrals, and educational information. They also promote public awareness through patient and health professional seminars, literature, and publicity campaigns. Their hope is to stimulate and support research to improve treatment and ultimately find the cause of and cure for scleroderma and related diseases.

Sjögren's Syndrome Foundation

http://www.sjogrens.org

Founded in 1983, the SSF provides patients with practical information and coping strategies that minimize the effects of Sjögren's. In addition, the foundation is the clearing house for medical information and is the recognized national advocate for Sjögren's. The foundation's mission is to educate patients and their families about Sjögren's, increase public and professional awareness of Sjögren's, and encourage research into new treatments and a cure.

Syndromes Without a Name USA

http://www.undiagnosed-usa.org

Syndromes Without a Name USA (SWAN USA) is a non-profit organization that offers support, information, and advice to families of children living with an undiagnosed syndrome, unknown diagnosis, or mystery diagnosis.

The Undiagnosed Disease Program

http://rarediseases.info.nih.gov

The Undiagnosed Diseases Program (UDP) is part of the NIH Common Fund initiative which focuses on the most puzzling medical cases at the NIH Clinical Center in Bethesda, Maryland. It was organized by the National Human Genome Research Institute (NHGRI), the NIH Office of Rare Diseases Research

(ORDR), and the NIH Clinical Center. Many medical specialties from other NIH research centers and institutes contribute the expertise needed to conduct the program, including endocrinology, immunology, oncology, dermatology, dentistry, cardiology, and genetics.

Government Resources and Financial Assistance

AbbVie Patient Assistance Foundation

http://www.abbviepaf.org

This foundation provides AbbVie medicines at no cost to people experiencing financial difficulties.

American Hospital Association: Patient Bill of Rights

http://www.aha.org

AHA's Patients' Bill of Rights brochure informs patients about what they should expect during their hospital stay with regard to their rights and responsibilities. The brochure is available in multiple languages.

Americans with Disabilities Act

http://www.ada.gov

This site educates readers on The Americans with Disabilities Act (ADA) which was signed into law on July 26, 1990 by President George H. W. Bush. The ADA is one of America's most comprehensive pieces of civil rights legislation that prohibits discrimination and guarantees that people with disabilities have the same opportunities as everyone else to enjoy employment opportunities, purchase goods and services, and to participate in state and local government programs and services. Modeled after the Civil Rights Act of 1964 (which prohibits discrimination on the basis of race, color, religion, sex, or national origin) and Section 504 of the Rehabilitation Act of 1973, the ADA is an "equal opportunity" law for people with disabilities.

Co-Pay Relief Program

http://www.copays.org

The Patient Advocate Foundation's (PAF) Co-Pay Relief Program (CPR) provides direct financial support to insured patients (including Medicare Part D beneficiaries) who are financially and medically qualified for pharmaceutical treatments and prescription medication co-payments, coinsurance, and deductibles relative to their diagnosis.

Disability.Gov

https://www.disability.gov

The site offers helpful resources on topics such as how to apply for disability benefits, find a job, get health care, or pay for accessible housing.

Patient Advocate Foundation

http://www.patientadvocate.org

Patient Advocate Foundation provides patients with arbitration, mediation, and negotiation support to settle issues with access to care, medical debt, and job retention related to their illness.

U.S. Department of Education

http://www2.ed.gov

Within the U.S. Department of Education, the Office for Civil Right's (OCR) mission is to ensure equal access to education through the enforcement of civil rights in schools. An important responsibility of the OCR is specifically to eliminate discrimination against students with disabilities.

U.S. Department of Health and Human Services: Mental Health

http://www.mentalhealth.gov

MentalHealth.gov aims to educate the general public, health and emergency preparedness professionals, policy makers, government and business leaders, school systems, and local communities about mental health.

United States Office of Social Security

http://www.ssa.gov/disabilityssi/

The Social Security and Supplemental Security Income disability programs are the largest of several Federal programs that help people with disabilities. While these two programs are different in many ways, both are administered by the Social Security Administration and only individuals who have a disability and meet medical criteria may qualify for benefits under either program.

For Caregivers

Caregiver Action Network (CAN)

http://www.caregiveraction.org

The Caregiver Action Network is the nation's leading family caregiver organization working to improve the quality of life for more than 65 million Americans who care for loved ones with chronic conditions, disabilities, disease, or the frailties of old age. CAN (formerly the National Family Caregivers Association) is a nonprofit organization providing education, peer support, and resources to family caregivers across the country free of charge. CAN serves a broad spectrum of family caregivers, ranging from the parents of children with special needs to the families and friends of wounded soldiers, from a young couple dealing with a diagnosis of MS to adult children caring for parents with Alzheimer's disease.

Today's Caregiver Magazine

http://www.caregiver.com

Caregiver Media Group is a leading provider of information, support and guidance for family and professional caregivers. Founded in 1995, they produce *Today's Caregiver* magazine, the first national magazine dedicated to caregivers and the Fearless Caregiver Conferences. Their website includes topic-specific newsletters, online discussion lists, back issue articles of *Today's Caregiver* magazine, chat rooms, and an online store. Caregiver Media Group and all of its products are developed for caregivers, about caregivers, and by caregivers.

Family Caregiver Alliance

https://www.caregiver.org

The Family Caregiver Alliance was the first community-based nonprofit organization in the country to address the needs of families and friends providing long-term care for loved ones at home. They illuminate the caregivers' daily challenges to better the lives of caregivers nationally, provide them the assistance they need and deserve, and champion their cause through education, services, research, and advocacy.

National Alliance for Caregiving

http://www.caregiving.org

Recognizing that family caregivers provide important societal and financial contributions toward maintaining the well-being of those they care for, the National Alliance for Caregiving's mission is to be an objective national resource on family caregiving with the goal of improving the quality of life for families and care recipients.

Pharmaceutical Companies

Abbot Laboratories

http://www.abbott.com

Alexion

http://alxn.com

Amicus

http://www.amicusrx.com

AstraZeneca

http://www.astrazeneca.com

Bayer

http://www.bayer.com

BioMarin

http://www.biomarin.com

Brystol-Myers Squib

http://www.bms.com

Centric Health Resources

http://www.centrichealthresources.com

Genzyme

http://www.genzyme.com

GlaxoSmithKline

http://www.gsk.com

Johnson & Johnson

https://www.jnj.com

Merck & Co

http://www.merck.com

Novartis

https://www.novartis.com

Pfizer

http://www.pfizer.com

Roche

http://www.roche.com

Sanofi

http://www.sanofi.us

Shire

http://www.shire.com

Sigma-Tau

http://www.sigmatau.com

Vertex

http://www.vrtx.com

Rare Disease Foundations

5p- Syndrome, Cat Cry Syndrome, Cri du Chat Syndrome

http://www.fivepminus.org

1p36 Deletion Syndrome

http://www.1p36dsa.org

22Q Deletion Syndrome

http://www.amp22q.org

22q11.2 Deletion Syndrome

http://www.22q11ireland.org

Aceruloplasminemia, Neurodegeneration with Brain Iron Accumulation Disorders, Hallervorden-Spatz Syndrome

http://www.nbiadisorders.org

Acid Maltase Deficiency, Pompe's Disease

http://www.amda-pompe.org

Acromegaly and Gigantism

http://www.acromegalycommunity.com

ADCY5 Mutation

http://www.adcy5.org

ADNP Syndrome, Helsmoortal Van Der AA Syndrome

http://www.adnpkids.com

Adrenal Insufficiency

http://www.aiunited.org

Adrenoleukodystrophy

http://www.aldconnect.org

http://www.aidanjackseegerfoundation.org

Adult Polyglucosan Body Disease

http://www.apbdrf.org

Alagille Syndrome

http://www.alagille.org

Alkaptonuria

http://www.akusociety.org

http://www.akusocietyna.org

Alpha-1 Antitrypsin Deficiency

http://www.alphaone.org

Alport Syndrome

http://www.alportsyndrome.org

Alström Syndrome

http://www.alstromangels.com

Alternating Hemiplegia of Childhood

http://www.ahckids.org

http://www.ahcfe.eu

Amyloidosis

http://www.amyloidosisresearchfoundation.org

http://www.arci.org

Amyloidosis Alect2

http://www.lect2.org

Aplastic Anemia, Myelodysplastic Syndromes, Paroxysmal Nocturnal Hemoglobinuria

http://www.aamds.org

APS Type 1 (APECED)

http://apstype1.org

Arachnoiditis

http://www.facebook.com/ArachnoiditisSocietyfor
AwarenessandPrevention

Arterial Tortuosity Syndrome

http://www.atwistoffate-ats.com

Ataxia-Telangiectasia

http://atcp.org

Atypical Hemolytic Uremic Syndrome

http://www.atypicalhus.net

Autoimmune Hepatitis

http://www.aihep.org

Bardet-Biedl Syndrome

http://www.bardetbiedl.org

Barth Syndrome

http://barthsyndrome.org

Batten Disease

http://www.beyondbatten.org

Behcet's Disease

http://www.behcets.com

Bohring-Opitz Syndrome

http://www.bos-foundation.org

Castleman Disease

http://www.castlemannetwork.org

Cavernous Angioma

http://www.angiomaalliance.org

Cerebral Autosomal Dominant Arteriopathy Subcortical Infarcts Leukoencephalopathy

http://cadasilassociation.org

Congenital Adrenal Hyperplasia

http://caresfoundation.org

Congenital Disorders of Glycosylation (CDG)

http://www.alphaepsilonomega.org/foundation/amour

Creatine Transport Deficiency, Guanidinoacetate Methyltransferase Deficiency, L-Arginine: Glycine Amidinotransferase

http://creatineinfo.org

Crohn's Disease, Ulcerative Colitis

http://www.crohnscolitisfoundation.org

Cryoglobulinemia

http://www.allianceforcryo.org

Cryopyrin-Associated Periodic Syndromes, Neonatal-Onset Multisystem Inflammatory Disease, Chronic Infantile Neurological Cutaneous and Articular Syndrome, Familial Cold Auto Inflammatory Syndrome

http://www.autoinflammatory.org

Cushing's Syndrome

http://www.csrf.net/

Cystic Fibrosis

http://www.cfri.org

Duchenne Muscular Dystrophy

http://www.coalitionduchenne.org

Duchenne Muscular Dystrophy, Becker Muscular Dystrophy

http://www.parentprojectmd.org

Dystonia

http://dystonia-foundation.org

Ehlers-Danlos Syndrome

http://www.edsers.com

http://www.ehlersdanlosnetwork.org

Eosinophilic Disorders

http://apfed.org

Epilepsy

http://www.epilepsywarriors.org

Fabry Disease

http://www.fabry.org

Familial Adenomatous Polyposis

http://www.hcctakesguts.org

Familia Exudative Vitreopothy (FEVR)

https://www.facebook.com/cailees.corner

Fibrodysplasia Ossificans Progressiva, Myositis Ossificans Progressiva

http://www.ifopa.org

Fibromuscular Dysplasia

http://www.fmdsa.org

Friedreichs Ataxia

http://www.curefa.org

Gaucher Disease

http://www.gaucherdisease.org

Glycogen Storage Disease

http://www.agsdus.org

Guillain-Barré Syndrome, Chronic Inflammatory Demyelinating Polyneuropathy

http://www.gbs-cidp.org

Hospital-Acquired Necrotizing Fasciitis

http://www.patientsafetyasap.org

Huntington's Disease

http://www.hdsa.org

Idiopathic Intracranial Hypertension

http://www.ihaveiih.com

Interstitial Lung Disease

http://www.child-foundation.com

Jacobsen Syndrome, 11q Chromosome

http://www.11qusa.org/home

Kabuki Syndrome

http://www.allthingskabuki.org

Klippel-Feil Syndrome

http://kfsalliance.org

Leukodystrophies

http://www.thecalliopejoyfoundation.org

Leukodystrophy

http://www.missionmassimo.com

Lynch Syndrome

http://lynchcancers.com

Lysosomal Diseases, India

http://www.lysosomaldiseasenetwork.org

Marfan Syndrome

http://www.marfan.org

Mayer-Rokitansky-Küster-Hauser Syndrome

http://www.beautifulyoumrkh.org

Metabolic Disorders

http://www.themetabolicfoundation.com

Multiple Endocrine Neoplasi

http://amensupport.org

Multiple Pediatric Rare Diseases

http://www.littlemisshannah.org

Multiple Rare Diseases

http://awareofangels.org

http://chivecharities.org

http://www.everylifefoundation.org

http://rarediseaseunited.org

http://sanfordresearch.org/cords

Multiple Rare Diseases, Undiagnosed

http://rareundiagnosed.org

Narcolepsy

http://www.narcolepsynetwork.org

http://www.wakeupnarcolepsy.org

Nemaline Myopathy

http://www.buildingstrength.org

Neurosarcoidosis, Sarcoidosis

http://www.sarcoidosisofli.com

Niemann Pick Disease

http://www.nnpdf.org

Niemann Pick Type C

http://addiandcassi.com

Ohtahara Syndrome

http://www.ohtahara.org

One or More Extra X and/or Y Chromosomes

http://www.genetic.org

Peyronie's Disease

http://www.peyroniesassociation.org

Phenylketonuria

http://www.npkua.org

Phenylketonuria and Allied Disorders

http://www.go-ipad.org

Pituitary Disorders

http://www.pituitary.org

Prader-Willi Syndrome, Abnormal Chromosome 15 (15q11-q13).

http://www.fpwr.org

RASopathy Syndromes

http://rasopathiesnet.org

Sanfilippo Syndrome

http://www.bensdream.org

http://www.curesff.org

Sanfilippo Syndrome, Mucopolysaccharidoses (MPSIII)

http://www.jonahsjustbegun.org

Sarcoidosis

http://www.stopsarcoidosis.org

Short Bowel Syndrome/Intestinal Failure

http://www.sbscure.org

Sickle Cell Disease

http://www.asapbeinformed.org

http://atlantascar.com

http://www.boldlipsforsicklecell.com

http://sc101.org

Skin Diseases, Ichthyosis

http://www.firstskinfoundation.org

SYNGAP1

http://www.bridgesyngap.org

Tuberous Sclerosis Complex

http://www.bcureful.org

Undiagnosed

http://www.undiagnosed-usa.org

Wolf-Hirschhorn Syndrome and Related 4p Conditions

http://www.4p-supportgroup.org

References

Ally, patient, in discussion with the author, November 2014.

Dawn Wiggins, licensed marriage and family therapist, in discussion with the author, February 2016, March 2016, February 2017.

Friedlander, J. 2012. *Business from Bed: The 6-Step Comeback Plan to Get Yourself Working After a Health Crisis.* New York: Demos Health Publishing.

Jacqueline, I. 2017. "Rare Diseases: Facts and Statistics." https://globalgenes.org/rare-diseases-facts-statistics.

Lauren Stiles, president and founder of Dysautonomia International, in discussion with the author, November 2014.

Paula Peena, mother of patient, in discussion with the author, March 2016, September 2016.

Shire Pharmaceutical. "Rare Disease Impact Report: Insights From Patients and the Medical Community." https://globalgenes.org/wp-content/uploads/2013/04/ShireReport-1.pdf.

Suris, J. C., P. A. Michaud, and R. Viner. 2004. "The Adolescent with a Chronic Condition. Part I: Developmental Issues." Accessed April 2017. https://www.ncbi.nlm.nih.gov/pmc/articles.

Travis Love, patient, in discussion with the author, November 2014.

Tricia Holderman, patient, in discussion with the author, November 2014.

Yang, Y. C., C. Boen, K. Gerken, T. Li, K. Schorpp, and K. M. Harris. 2015. "Social Relationships and Physiological Determinants of Longevity Across the Human Life Span." *PNAS* 113(3): 578–83.

Ilana Jacqueline is author of the award-winning blog *Let's Feel Better*. She started the blog at age twenty-two to share her humbling, hilarious, and heartfelt experiences coping with chronic illness. From full-contact fights with skull-cramping migraines to making peace with being a human pincushion, she writes boldly and unabashedly about breaking down, getting back up, and pulling off the bandage that is "coming out" about the shame and frustration of living with chronic illness.

Jacqueline is a health journalist and professional patient advocate whose work has included writing for publications like *Cosmopolitan* and *The Huffington Post* on the patient experience, as well as working for health care companies and patient advocacy groups as a consultant and advisor. She has a personal connection with the patient community, as she has been a patient with complex chronic illnesses throughout her life, including immune deficiency, dysautonomia, gastroparesis, and an adhesion disorder.

As a health advocate and regularly interviewed expert on chronic illness, Jacqueline looks to help patients advocate for themselves at their most vulnerable moments. She is currently working on multiple projects to help connect chronically ill patients with remote employment opportunities, financial and emotional support, as well as creating new programs for patient empowerment and awareness efforts. Jacqueline lives with her biochemist husband and literally the cutest apricot poodle you've ever seen in Boca Raton, FL.

MORE BOOKS *from*
NEW HARBINGER PUBLICATIONS

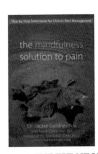
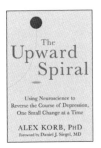
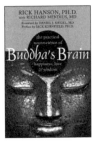
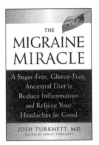
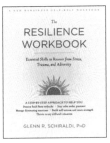
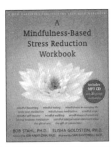
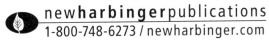

Register your **new harbinger** titles for additional benefits!

When you register your **new harbinger** title—purchased in any format, from any source—you get access to benefits like the following:

- Downloadable accessories like printable worksheets and extra content

- Instructional videos and audio files

- Information about updates, corrections, and new editions

Not every title has accessories, but we're adding new material all the time.

Access free accessories in 3 easy steps:

1. Sign in at NewHarbinger.com (or **register** to create an account).

2. Click on **register a book**. Search for your title and click the **register** button when it appears.

3. Click on the **book cover or title** to go to its details page. Click on **accessories** to view and access files.

That's all there is to it!

If you need help, visit:

NewHarbinger.com/accessories

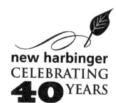

new harbinger
CELEBRATING
40 YEARS